FACING ADVERSITY

Words That Heal

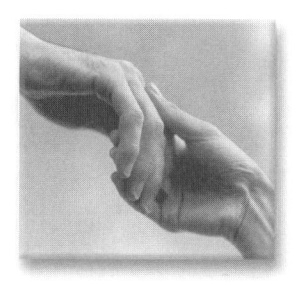

Herbert L. Gravitz, Ph.D.

Healing Visions Press
Santa Barbara, California

FACING ADVERSITY
Words That Heal

By Herbert L. Gravitz, Ph.D.

All rights reserved. No part of this book may be reproduced or transmitted, except as part of a book review or similar project, without written permission from the publisher.

This book is not a substitute for psychological, medical, legal, financial or other professional services. If expert counseling or guidance is needed, the services of a competent professional should be sought.

Copyright ©2004 by Herbert L. Gravitz, Ph.D.

Healing Visions Press, Santa Barbara, California
www.HealTheFamily.com

ISBN: 0-96611046-3

Publisher's Cataloging-in-Publications
(Provided by *Quality Books, Inc.*)

Gravitz, Herbert L., 1942-
    Facing adversity: words that heal / Herbert L. Gravitz
    p. cm.
    Includes bibliographical references.
LCCN 2003112565
ISBN: 0-96611046-3

    1. Healing—Psychological aspects. 2. Sick—Family relationships. 3. Mental healing. 4. Soul—Psychological aspects.   I. Title

    R726.5.G73 2004   615.5
                       QBI33-1631

Edited by Gail M. Kearns, To Press and Beyond, Santa Barbara, California

Cover and book design by
Peri Poloni, Knockout Design, www.knockoutbooks.com

Printed in United States

Dedication

*To Leslie Ann Wilcove Gravitz,
the love of my life*

Other Books by Herbert L. Gravitz

Mental Illness and the Family: Unlocking the Doors to Triumph.
Santa Barbara, California: Healing Visions Press, 2004.

Obsessive Compulsive Disorder: New Help for the Family.
Santa Barbara, California: Healing Visions Press, 1998.

Genesis: Spirituality in Recovery from Childhood Traumas (with J. Bowden).
Pompano Beach, Florida: Health Communications, Inc., 1988.

Recovery: A Guide for Adult Children of Alcoholics (with J. Bowden).
New York, New York: Simon and Schuster, 1987.

Forthcoming Books

Bittersweet: Cancer as a Sacred Wound.
Santa Barbara, California: Healing Visions Press, 2005.

Trauma and Adversity: Triumph's Crucible.
Santa Barbara, California: Healing Visions Press, 2005.

Contents

A Word From the Author	vii
Preface: A Word About Words	xi
Introduction	xv
CHAPTER 1: **The Beginning**	1
CHAPTER 2: **The Problem**	13
CHAPTER 3: **The Diagnoses**	41
CHAPTER 4: **The Wound**	63
CHAPTER 5: **The Impact of the Wound**	81
CHAPTER 6: **Sacred and Profane Wounds**	101
CHAPTER 7: **The Journey**	135
CHAPTER 8: **The Method**	159
CHAPTER 9: **Refamilying**	201
CHAPTER 10: **The Outcome**	245
CHAPTER 11: **Summary**	267
Postscript	291
About the Author	295
Partial List of Contributors	299
Contributor Index	309
Subject Index	317

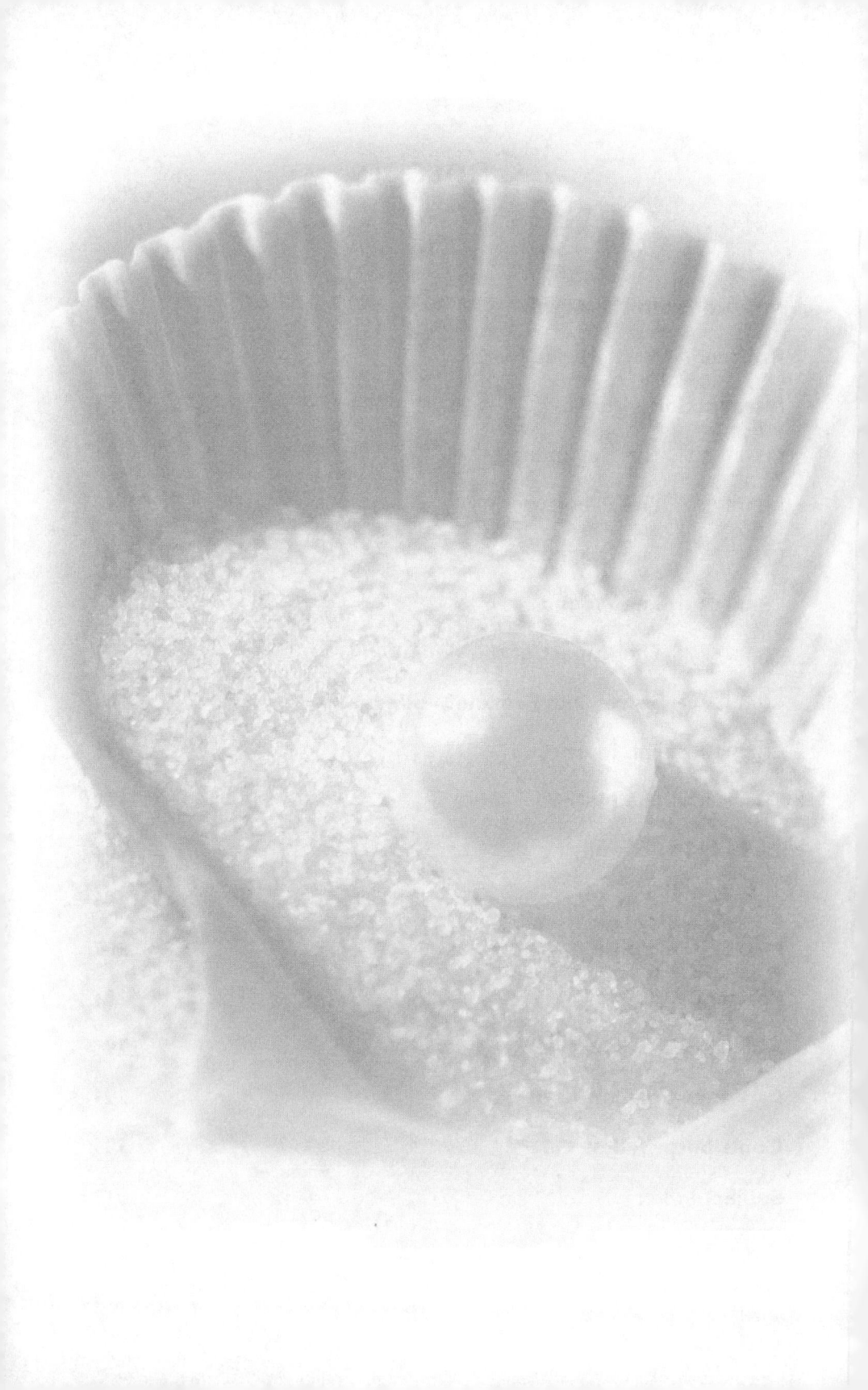

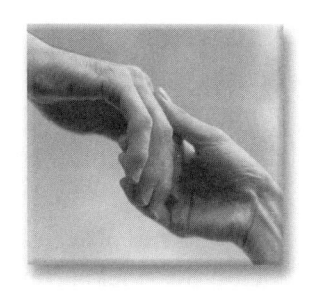

A Word From the Author

Welcome to what I anticipate can be a highly useful operator's manual for navigating our brave new world. We now inhabit a world of emergencies, crises, other stresses, and events that exceed our usual and customary ways of coping—in short, a world of ever-increasing complexity and adversity, particularly in the wake of September 11, 2001. Facing adversity with hope, courage, compassion, equanimity, and a loving heart, ennobling the finest qualities we human beings possess, is the challenge of our time as we live in a world characterized by unprecedented turmoil and change.

On every front, from the horrors of global war to the alarms of a sagging global economy, we face not only the potential extinction of the human race but also the actual extinction of untold species of animals and plants that occur on a daily basis. All life forms are facing adversities at a more accelerating and frightening pace than at any other time in history. While some tribulations are clearly more serious and devastating than others, each of us must deal with one hardship or another with increasing frequency.

Now is the time both to recognize the turmoil of our times and to understand what advanced civilizations of all times have known:

namely, adversity is the soil from which triumph springs. We must remember that life's meaning is often made clearer by our misfortunes. From those misfortunes, a mission can emerge that can alter our life in the direction of bringing out our finest qualities and truest nature.

A man recently diagnosed with the physical disease of cancer, in addition to suffering from the mental illness of schizophrenia, explained facing the unexpected and dreaded in the following way, words that have always stayed with me. He said, "Emergencies are now commonplace, and the best way to view an emergency is my opportunity to 'emerge-and-see.'"

There are many different kinds of adversities. While not entirely inclusive, the major adversities and emergencies that we face can be seen as three in number:

- Traumas, whether physical, mental, emotional, spiritual, environmental, economic, or more likely a combination—traumas can be of human origin, such as abuse, or of natural origin, such as an earthquake or hurricane

- Illnesses, whether physical, mental, or more commonly both—illnesses can be of sudden onset or linger for decades, gradually stealing the life of both the person with the illness and his or her loved ones

- Addictions, whether from alcohol or other drugs, as well as addictions to food, work, or even sex.

To make matters even worse, addictions frequently accompany and are present in the aftermath of illness and trauma. Virtually all adversities stem from one or a combination of these three. As we have seen, adversities are inescapable.

Fortunately, we already have a map that charts the journey from surviving to thriving. It is both as old as time, revealed in the ancient scriptures and texts, and as new as today's state-of-the-art science and technology. Both are being shown to reveal the same messages to enable us to transform life's horrors to sources of awareness and appreciation for life's moments.

In this timely collection of some of the most inspiring, beautiful, and empowering words from the greatest thinkers of all times, you will be introduced to opportunities to 'emerge and see,' regardless of the type of trauma, illness, or addiction. Optimistic in tone and practical in application, this is a book for everyone who faces a life-changing adversity, for it illustrates the steps toward healing and recovery through which individuals and their loved ones pass as they face and overcome the obstacles that life invariably presents.

By reading the healing words spoken by ancient and modern sages, mystics, scholars, and scientists, you can directly learn the attitudes, feelings, thoughts, and behaviors taught by the masters throughout the ages. By providing new pathways, these words consistently show how to surmount the challenges from any of life's major wounding events and assaults.

Words That Heal is an invitation for you to claim or reclaim your inherent, natural drive to make sense of your experience and move forward toward a more universal and encompassing vision of life. Experience the principles to guide you to a full and well-lived life, regardless of the circumstances in which you may find yourself.

Unlike most books, this is a book that can be easily read a few minutes at a time by today's busy, on-the-go wisdom seeker. The journey is simpler than you may imagine and only awaits the serious traveler.

Wise words, by their very nature, are repeated and shared often. Thus, despite my best efforts, it's quite possible in this book that someone other than the originator of a quotation may be credited or that changes in the original quote may appear. The wisdom of the words, however, is unmistakable.

Godspeed on the journey, your journey, from surviving adversities to thriving in spite of—or more to the point, because of—them.

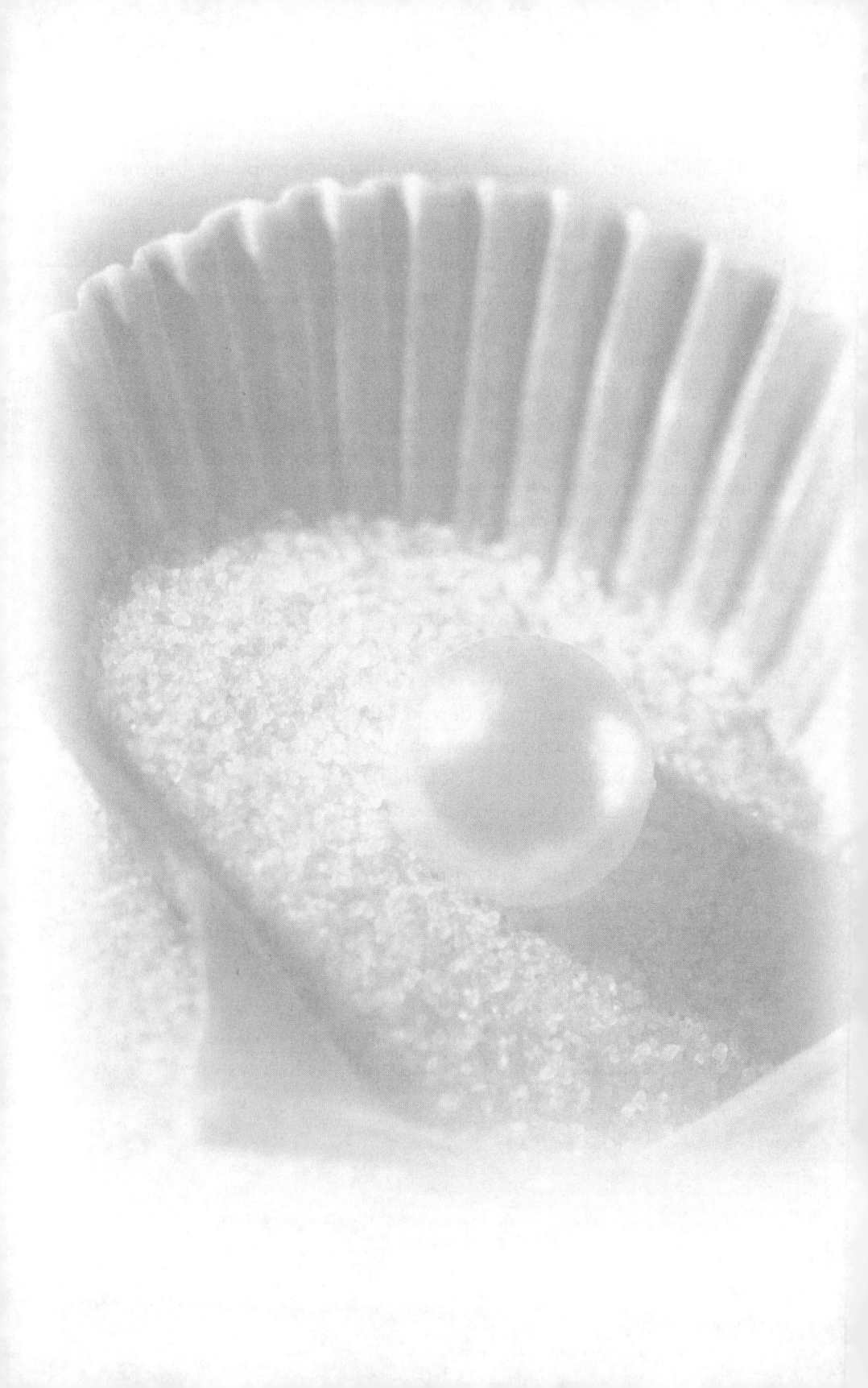

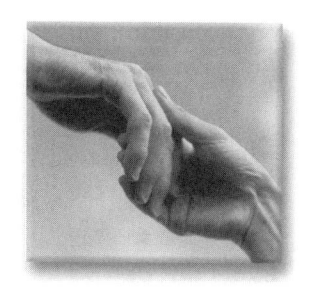

Preface: A Word About Words

Words can be magical, often providing us with the wisdom and strength to transcend the most harsh and difficult of life's circumstances. More than two thousand years ago, the great Roman orator and statesman, Cicero, suggested the use of "healing words," *iatroi logoi,* for those who sought counsel and consolation from life's greatest problems.

Words are not just sounds or written symbols; they are the vital forces that give us the power to convey, communicate, and share our very thoughts and feelings. It is through words that we express ourselves, as well as give meaning and substance to our everyday experience. In fact, they are godly, as the following words that open the book of John in the New Testament of the Bible attest: "In the beginning was the Word, and the Word was with God, and the Word was God."

The power of words lies in their ability to be catalysts for growth, catapulting us to new ways of viewing our circumstance and, ultimately, ourselves. In addition, the enchantment of the right words often fosters the attitudes, feelings, thoughts, and behaviors that we need in order to embrace every challenge as the opportunity that it can be.

A few well-timed and well-placed words can mean the difference between triumph or defeat, happiness or sadness, perspective or confusion—and, at times, even life or death. Because life is a contest of opposites, words become one of the most important mediums through which we make sense of it.

What is more, words form a powerful container that hold our beliefs. They give birth to our beliefs, and it is our beliefs that become the filters through which we see and make sense of the world. Yet, most of us would be amazed by how arbitrary, automatic, and unconscious our words and beliefs are. Unfolding through a reciprocal dance, our inner beliefs interact with the outside world of circumstance, as we craft much of our interpretation of reality through the use of words.

By understanding the role of beliefs, whether acquired through experience, readings, or the stories we tell ourselves, we may participate in the construction of a world that helps us create the realities we desire. Because beliefs are constructed interpretations of a situation and the meaning or meanings that we give the situation, they are instrumental in determining what we see and don't see.

But where can we find the beliefs to guide us to a life fulfilled? Where are the words that can lead us to a life worth having and losses worth enduring? And where are the truths that have withstood the test of time, applying now as well as they did when they were first expressed? These everlasting truths are "eternal truths." They are eternal precisely because their value and meaning have withstood the test of time. Indeed, they are found in the writings and sayings of the wisdom teachers of all ages and times.

These timeless and everlasting truths are locked away either in texts most of us will never see, or they are collected by other keepers of wisdom. This is why collections of sayings and quotes, gathered from ancient to modern times, are a time-honored tradition.

The words that soothe life's greatest problems, however, are rarely found in a neat, systematic, or organized manner that is specifically designed to illustrate the fundamental principles and rules for triumphing over and healing from life's major difficulties. The adversities of illness, addiction, and trauma are life's greatest problems, and they rarely occur by themselves, which means that when one is present, the others are often not far behind.

As you will find thoughout the pages that follow, words can form a map to the great truths, bringing calm to the lives of those who experience illness, addiction, and other trauma. Consequently, words are among our most powerful tools for healing the human condition. The mindful, careful, and thoughtful use of words facilitates human progress, and never before have we so needed the words that can heal us, our country, and our planet.

The healing words in this book can allow you to shift your mind, body, and spirit to a state of consciousness in which you can more easily choose grace and ease rather than addiction and *dis-ease*. Helping you to redefine and expand the meaning of the pains and hurts that keep you hostage to any major adversity, this book can enable you to move beyond the limits of a narrowed mind, injured body, and disquieted spirit.

Not surprisingly, science has shown the remarkable power of words. Researchers have now demonstrated that genetic shifts in the actual sequence of the DNA molecule—the inner core of our cells that restores and repairs the essence of our being—may be facilitated by thoughts, feelings, and emotions, all of which are mediated by the words that form our beliefs. Further, quantum science is showing that emotion, often elicited by the use of words, can be a switch to trigger specific DNA codes within the body, codes that foster health or sickness.

Modern science, of course, is only confirming what ancient knowledge has shown all along. Proverbs 16:24 says, "Encouraging words are as honey/Sweet to the soul and health to the being." The strength of words is echoed in the words of Saint Theresa of Lisieux, one of the most widely loved saints of the Roman Catholic Church who lived from 1873-1897. Affectionately known as "the Little Flower," she said, "Words lead to deeds.... They prepare the soul, make it ready, and move it to tenderness."

So, dear reader, become ready to be moved. All that you may need to be inspired, to be healed, and to triumph follows. Paradoxically, nothing may be new and everything can change. Allow the eternal truths in an ever-changing universe to reveal inner values and provide counsel for outer situations.

You can find startling statements throughout these pages. One of the most helpful may be to realize that the struggles in your life are not the problem. They are not indications of something wrong, but rather evidence of an emerging solution, for it is natural for us to struggle as we discover and create the meaning of our lives. Know that as you acknowledge your struggles, you unlock the doors to your solutions. You need adversity to triumph. The second may be the realization that paradox is one of the pillars through which one must pass on his or her way to enlightenment.

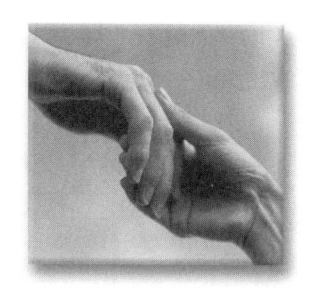

Introduction

Allow me to introduce myself. I am a clinical psychologist with a private practice in Santa Barbara, California, an author of other books and professional articles on healing and recovery, a workshop and seminar leader, and an ardent student of illness, addiction, and other traumas. When I present lectures to both professional and non-professional audiences, I often half-kiddingly say that I have earned two doctorate degrees in psychology. The first I acquired when I was six years old from the "school of hard knocks," as my father used to call life. I majored in grief counseling, I minored in trauma, and my primary client was my family, especially my mother, whose entire family was murdered in the Nazi Holocaust. I received the second Ph.D. when I was twenty-six from the University of Tennessee. It was by far the easier of the two!

Since I was six years old, I have wanted to become skilled at how to heal the family. Today, I am still learning how to heal the family. But now I have more knowledge, more support, and the permission to heal my own wounds. Like most of us, I have incurred many wounds after six decades of living. While the trauma of the Holocaust has formed an ever-present backdrop to my life, I have also personally suffered major illness, minor illness, major loss, including the deaths of both of my parents and people central in my life, as well as other adversities.

It is *because of* these injuries, not *in spite of* them, that I feel especially graced and enjoy more freedom today than ever before. While my own personal odyssey of wounding has not been an easy one, it has been more than worthwhile. It has forged the person I am today, and I have learned to like and respect myself when at one time I didn't. The renowned mythologist Joseph Campbell once said, "The privilege of a lifetime is being who you are." Nothing can be truer for the person who has made the transition from survivor to thriver of life's difficulties.

What is often not said, however, is how much work this shift takes and how hard this heroic journey is. We need many provisions for this odyssey, especially sound maps to guide us. The words in the form of messages that are contained in *Words That Heal,* when read deliberately and intentionally, maximize the formation of new thoughts and beliefs that can shape in positive ways your experience or reality. What is more, the words in this book can help you open the doors to triumph over and recover from virtually any of life's major injuries, whether illness, addiction, or other trauma. They are assembled for you so that you can begin to use the power they contain from the first page forward.

Words That Heal seeks to organize the basic principles of healing and triumph needed by families under the influence of major adversity by serving as a compendium of some of the most inspiring and moving words in print today. This book is also written to serve as a companion book to *Recovery: A Guide for Adult Children of Alcoholics; Obsessive Compulsive Disorder: New Help for the Family*; and *Mental Illness and the Family: Unlocking the Doors to Triumph.* All three of my previous books mirror and link the words, the principles, and the eternal truths that are presented in this book.

These words that heal are expressed in many different ways. They appear in parables, wise sayings, quips, psalms, proverbs, precepts, dictums, aphorisms, truisms, adages, axioms, maximums, and paradoxes. Some of these words of healing are solemn; some are humorous. Some are recent in origin, some not so recent, and others come from antiquity.

Some words are from scientists and artists, while others are from philosophers and healers. Some are words that have just "popped out of my mouth" as I have worked with clients, while others have been uttered by my own family, friends, and the families whom I have been privileged to know. Still others are the words of health professionals who describe key terms and concepts unique to their work. There are even a few that come from a Chinese fortune cookie or two. Some are even displayed on bumper stickers. (Because not all of the sayings are gender sensitive, however, please do not allow the overuse of the male pronoun *he* or the noun *man* to deter your learning or enjoyment.)

All of these words that heal, which convey beliefs that can change your life, have profound meaning for me, and I have been gathering them, and savoring them, for almost five decades. They have inspired me and given me direction and comfort when there seemed little. They have also grounded me in realities of possibility, especially when I have been tired, stressed, or overwhelmed.

I cannot always walk my talk. I often stumble on my own words, slipping into periods of unconsciousness and victimization, as well as regret and blame. Nevertheless, I now have learned where the path resides. When I am lost or humbled by yet another of life's many "growth opportunities," which almost always seem to be some extraordinary or overwhelmingly painful experience, I remember the trail.

This trail resembles the ancient trials of the heroes of the past. At a time in history when we need more heroes, not fewer, it is becoming more and more up to each of us to step into the shoes of heroism, for there is much around us that requires heroic actions. The morsels of wisdom from the sages of all times line this trail. They deal not just with surviving life, but actually thriving *in the midst of* illness, addiction, and other trauma, unlocking the doors to triumphing over any of life's adversities, calamities, and misfortunes.

When I have shared these sayings with families, whether in my consultation room, in lectures, or in workshops, I have been told repeatedly how helpful they have been for *every* member of the family in his or her ongoing struggle toward healing and triumph. They apply to both the person directly afflicted by adversity (that is, "the primary sufferer") and the family, loved ones, and the friends, who are directly and indirectly affected (that is, "the secondary sufferers"). I have referred to these secondary sufferers as "the neglected affected" in prior writings.

And in my prior writings, I have stressed my clinical observation that it is often *after* each family member has begun to attend to his or her own unique problems and issues that the family as a whole can heal and triumph. When making family interaction the *starting point* of healing, my experience has been that progress is impeded because each and every member of the family has his and her own story to tell first. Until this story is told and witnessed, healing is limited. Yet, paradoxically, the same words can help every member of the family, whether the primary or secondary sufferer.

I have considered many different ways to share these healing and inspiring words that can help every family member. Because they have been so valuable to those with whom I work as well as to me personally, I wanted to present them in the very ways that I originally heard or read them—right from "the horse's mouth," so to speak. I thought of arranging them in a linear sequence—some at the beginning and some at the end, sort of like a continuum toward healing. This led to grouping them into categories.

Seeing patterns emerge, I finally decided that they could be most helpful to you if they followed, however loosely, the stages of recovery that I have described in my writings and talks—like a kind of "surround sound" to accompany the stages and transitions of triumph and healing. A friend who read a draft of this book called them "sound bytes for the soul." So, I present this collage of healing words to you, my reader, in the hope that you may find comfort, strength, and direction from them, just as so many others have with whom I have worked.

The unique feature of this particular collection is the use of carefully selected words woven throughout the stages of healing from illness, addiction, and other traumas that I have witnessed firsthand in my clinical practice for more than three decades. For within these words is a story, a story as old as time and as timely as now. It is the story of growing up and growing through all of life's events. The words chosen to tell this story are those words spoken directly by the world's greatest and wisest, whether past or present. A coherent story not just for surviving but actually thriving in life is revealed. Ageless, it is the same story that ancient texts describe and modern science is proving.

After a preparatory chapter sets the tone for the experiences you can encounter on your healing journey, chapter 2 presents statements of "the problem" that faces us through a host of incisive sayings and eye-opening statistics relating to life's major difficulties. Chapter 3 follows with the importance of an accurate diagnosis and assessment of the situation, which lets you know what you could be up against. Next, in chapters 4 and 5 respectively, I present words that relate to the wounding inherent in the problem(s) itself and the impact of this wounding on others. Chapter 6 develops the critical distinction between "profane" and "sacred" wounds that *all* those who are injured can immediately find helpful. Sayings describing the journey of healing are presented in chapter 7, and inspiring words about the methods, or ways to achieve healing and triumph, are presented in chapter 8. This leads to collections of sayings in chapter 9 that reflect what I have called "refamilying," or the coming together of the family after a wound's wake. Chapter 10 describes some of the benefits or outcomes you can expect when you allow yourself to come under the influence of healing words and the beliefs that they convey. I summarize salient points in the healing process in chapter 11. After this summary, I present a brief postscript. A partial list of contributors and two indexes, one by contributors and one by subjects, conclude the book.

Some quotes and sayings could apply to more than one chapter, or even might be better placed in a different grouping than I chose. There was, at times, a certain arbitrariness in selecting the expressions that accompanied each chapter. But the overriding concern was always *which* sayings and *which* words would serve you best, not *where* they most belonged.

I have also included a number of different sayings that suggest essentially similar points. I have intentionally done so for several reasons. Because repetition is the key to mastery, the more and varied the ways you read the same principle, the better. Also, different expressions of related points may speak more directly to some readers than to others. In addition, when one appreciates how the wisdom keepers throughout all of time have said virtually identical things, the universality of these truths becomes more evident, and the principles that underlie them become more useful and easily seen.

While the vast majority of sayings are non-technical and "user friendly," I also decided to include a small number of technical terms, such as definitions of some of the mental disorders from *DSM-IV* (the *Diagnostic and Statistical Manual of the American Psychiatric Association*), which is often referred to as the official "bible" of psychiatric diagnosis. I also have chosen to use terms and definitions from the literatures of relevant professional fields. For those who want a little taste of what the "pros" in the fields of illness, addiction, and trauma are saying, there are enough references to satisfy your appetite for more scientific information. And for those who find these a distraction, they can be easily skipped without interfering with the flow or continuity of the book.

It is important to note that while I am using the lens of illness, addiction, and other traumas *in general* to illustrate healing from a wide variety of mental, emotional, physical, and spiritual conditions, other severe, chronic, and persistent circumstances, such as poverty or prejudice, could just as well be described or emphasized. The universalization of life's insults has been known forever, and that knowledge can assuage the personal feelings of affront that so many of us feel. One of the greatest psychologists of modern times, Dr. Carl R. Rogers, reminds us: "The most personal [about us] is the most general."

Go slowly when you read these words—very slowly. Pause. Reflect. Become quiet. Don't just read them: ponder them. Live with them. Pick up the book often. More importantly, put it down often. Stop reading it after each passage or entry. Underline or star those that speak to *you*. Come back often to your favorite expressions. It can get tedious to read saying after saying unless you stop, think, reflect, meditate, and figure out where in *your* life you can tap into the words of some of our greatest sages, saints, mystics, and scientists. Only in this way can you acquire some of the resources that *you* may need to deal with *your* particular situation, or this leg of *your* journey. Allow yourself to be inspired, for inspiration is the source of all meaningful action, as is perspiration. And allow yourself to *feel* the wisdom of time and to be moved in the deepest recesses of your heart, mind, and soul.

To empower the words, it will be helpful to consciously, actively, and out loud, in your own voice, thank yourself for giving yourself the opportunity to heal. Thank yourself for giving yourself the chance to grow and develop beyond old and destructive patterns that hurt you and those you love.

Actively means right *now*. Can you literally take a moment… stop reading…pause…let yourself be trance-ported to a special place within, and simply take in the comfort for giving yourself this opportunity? It would be a wonder-full start.

Personally, I have certain expressions memorized, and I repeat them daily and even more often when I need them. Some are posted on my bathroom mirror, refrigerator door, or the dashboard of my car. One of my favorites is a statement my father often made. I can still hear his voice. In his European accent, he would say, "Herb, always remember—God gives you gifts and they are usually wrapped in problems." Then, with a twinkle in his eyes, he would add, "And you have to unwrap them before they are yours." Given that I, like you, am not immune to problems, the universality and the self-evident truths of these words have always been soothing and comforting, enabling me to go through my dark nights of the soul.

These sayings represent just a portion of the collective wisdom that we have acquired. While far from inclusive, they can give you enough of a taste of the wisdom of the ages to make an enormous difference in your (and your family's) life. Though they are simple assertions of truth, they make the truth that you know more fully available and understandable. One family member expressed this point in the following way: "These words are so obvious. Why couldn't I think of them myself?"

May the words gathered in this book inspire and comfort you in times of joy and sorrow, enabling you and your loved ones to find the meaning and relevance that can transform your traumas and disappointments into triumphs and trials that rival the heroic exploits and quests of our ancestors.

Blessings!

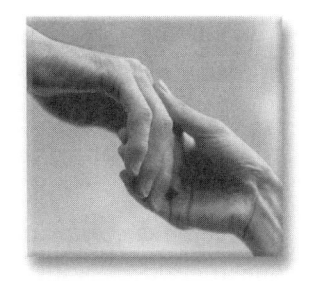

CHAPTER 1

The Beginning

If you, a family member, or a loved one are under or have just come under the influence of one of life's major or recurrent problems, whether a serious illness, addiction, or other trauma, you are about to take a journey—often, an exceedingly long and difficult one. Not only has your loved one's life been turned upside down, but *your* life most probably has as well. Many adjustments will need to be made by you, as major parts of your life may need to be reconsidered. And because adversity is rarely just an event, but rather a long-term process of adaptation and accommodation, your life may continue to change at an ever increasing, sometimes frightening, and often accelerating pace.

Your whole way of life may be altered: your daily routine, your sense of peace and quiet, your circle of friends, your privacy, your freedom, and your overall enjoyment and appreciation for life may change radically. You may lose the opportunity to see your child graduate from school, be present at your child's wedding, have grandchildren, experience a mutually satisfying relationship with a mate, receive an early retirement (or any retirement for that matter), or lose the chance for a host of other memorable occasions. Instead, you may spend long hours taking care of a loved one, even when he or she is being unkind and unappreciative.

You may have physical, emotional, mental, spiritual, and even financial burdens, where you once may have had none.

Like it or not, ready or not, with the ravages of serious illness, addiction, or other traumas, you and your loved one may have come to the end of one path, only to start another, one that is often more unclear and confusing. More to the point, both you and your loved one are experiencing a life transition; you are not merely experiencing a change in your circumstance. While many people use change and transition synonymously, there is value in distinguishing them.

A change is a situational shift. As agents from the outside that revolve around particular circumstances, change requires little internal reorganization. For example, you move into a new house; you buy a new car; you get a different job; you receive a promotion. None of these events typically require major modifications in your view of the world.

On the other hand, transitions are internal shifts and involve modifications in a person's perception of his or her meaning of events. It is not so much the changes in our life that we so resist or fear. It is the transitions, the doors that become closed or opened by the changes, for it is the transitions that involve the process of letting go of the old and ushering in the new. In between the letting go of the old and the taking hold of the new, there is invariably a period of chaos when things aren't the same way anymore. But they aren't the new way yet either.

While we focus on the outcome with change, the starting point for transition is the closing that we must make in order to leave the old situation behind. While change concerns events, transitions involve passages from one time to another. Passages always begin with the end of something, often something very precious. We proceed through a space of limbo, or uncertainty, which is often called "the dark night of the soul" by mystics, poets, and philosophers.

This three-phase process—ending, chaos, and beginning again—is what is meant by the term transition. Transitions are not designed to be easy and they are almost always challenging. They are the psychospiritual process people go through to come to terms with the new change. They involve going through phases of *adjusting* to changes. Transitions, therefore, presuppose adjustments. Living under the influence of ongoing adversity requires a transition; it is not simply a change from one state to another.

An old saying asserts that to enter the Temple of Enlightenment we have to pass through two pillars: the pillar of paradox and the pillar of confusion. Like all that is sacred, transitions can be full of paradox and confusion. For instance, there is the paradox that transitions always end with a new beginning.

Like the heroes of old who were called upon to save the kingdom, few of us request the confusion and paradox inherent in transitions. Like those who have come before us, we often don't want transitions; yet, we have little choice about their occurrence. Thus, we don't ask for illness; we don't ask for injuries; we don't ask for endings, or new beginnings. It is of little matter, however. A familiar joke states, people plan and God laughs.

Few of us are prepared for any losses that life brings upon us, let alone the big ones. Yet the sages and mystics of all times remind us that we seldom venture forward in life unless, metaphorically speaking, it is to "save the kingdom," or to find the precious thing(s) which we have grievously lost. As one of my clients said: "We don't wake up one morning when everything is going well and decide to go on the journey of a lifetime, one that will take us to the depths of our soul and the farthest reaches of our spirit." Extreme situations, such as illness, addiction, and other trauma, can bring out the worst in us—or they can bring out the best. Virtually all of us have a choice about how we use our desperation, but we don't seem to have a choice about whether we encounter distressing circumstances.

There are many ways, of course, to proceed on the voyage of healing and recovery: we can go kicking and screaming, lamenting our plight, or we can surrender to what lies in front of us, accepting whatever is ahead. We can decry the quest as a major detour to accomplishing our goals and satisfying our needs, or we can recognize—usually on faith—that regardless of the circumstance in which we find ourselves, the quest is the next superhighway leading us toward a meaningful and full life. In ancient days, problems, or trials as they were called, led to an initiation into a different and often higher level of consciousness and reality. They were to be expected.

The way you deal with the path is yours as a choice. So, let us proceed forward to new beginnings, those that can usher in opportunities for triumph, healing, rebirth, and growth. As we shall continue to discover, like the ancient heroes who came before us, we must first cross a threshold to behold a new beginning.

Come to the edge, he said.
They said: We are afraid.
Come to the edge, he said.
He pushed them...And they flew.

—*Guillaume Apollinaire*

... renewal comes neither by taking a rest nor changing the scenery, nor by adding something new to our lives, but by ending whatever is, and then entering a temporary state of chaos when everything is up for grabs and anything is possible. Then—but only then—can we come out of what is really a death-and-rebirth process with a new identity, a new sense of purpose, and a new store of life energy.

—*William Bridges*

Chapter 1: The Beginning

Every exit is an entry somewhere else.
—*Tom Stoppard*

Beginnings are always messy.
—*John Galsworthy*

Winning starts with beginning.
—*Bumper sticker*

The only joy in the world is to begin.
—*Cesare Pavese*

And to make an end is to make a beginning.
The end is where we start from.
—*T. S. Eliot*

One doesn't discover new lands without consenting to lose sight of the shore for a very long time.
—*André Gide*

I couldn't tell if that was the light at the end of the tunnel or the light of an oncoming train.
—*Family member*

Every beginning is a consequence.
Every beginning ends something.

—Paul Valery

Great is the art of beginning,
but greater the art of ending.

—Henry Wadsworth Longfellow

The end of a path is the beginning of another.

—Navaho proverb

When old words die out on the tongue,
new melodies break forth from the heart;
and where the old tracks are lost,
new country is revealed with its wonders.

—Rabindranath Tagore

Confusion is a word we have invented for an order
which is not yet understood.

—Henry Miller

An adventure is only an inconvenience rightly understood.
An inconvenience is only an adventure wrongly understood.

—G. K. Chesterton

Chapter 1: The Beginning

Transition helps you come to terms with change. It reorients you so that you can mobilize your energy to deal successfully with your new situation—whether it is a 'good' one or a 'bad' one doesn't matter—instead of being hampered by attitudes and behaviors that were developed for and more appropriate to your old situation…. It involves relinquishing the old habits and expectations and developing new ones that fit the new situation.

—*William Bridges*

Do not pray for an easy life;
Pray for greater strength.
Do not pray for tasks equal to your powers;
Pray for powers equal to your tasks.
Then the doing of your work shall be no miracle;
But you will be a miracle.
Every day you will wonder at yourself;
At the riches of the life that has come to you by the grace of God.
Faith is walking to the edge of all you have
And taking one more step.

—*Anonymous*

Through loyalty to the past, our mind refuses to realize that tomorrow's joy is possible only if today's makes way for it; that each wave owes the beauty of its line only to the withdrawal of the receding one.

—*André Gide*

Faith is to believe in what we do not see;
and the reward of this faith is to see what we believe.

—*St. Augustine*

Events are always in flux. One day people love you; the next day you're their target. One day a situation is running smoothly; the next day chaos reigns. One day you feel like you're an okay person; the next day you feel like you're an utter failure. These changes in life are always going to happen; they're part of the human experience. What we can change, however, is how we perceive. And that shift in our perception is a miracle.

—*Marianne Williamson*

Life does not accommodate you, it shatters you.
It is meant to, and it couldn't do it better.
Every seed destroys its container
or else there would be no fruition.

—*Florida Scott-Maxwell*

Cancer is okay if you like beginnings. Every day I have a new beginning. Every day I exchange who I thought I was for who I am now. I thought I was healthy; now I have cancer. I thought I had a treatable local recurrence; now it is most likely incurable metastatic cancer.... Today my body feels strong and pain-free; in a month I may have the torture of chemotherapy. Today I'm a vigorous and involved grandmother who likes to take her grandchildren to Disneyland; next year I may be a grandmother who mostly looks on and delights in her grandchildren by watching and listening to them.

—*Mondi Bridges*

I respect faith, but doubt is what gets you an education.

—*Wilson Mizner*

Chapter 1: The Beginning

> What the caterpillar calls the end of life,
> the master calls a butterfly.
>
> —*Richard Bach*

> An era can be said to end
> when its basic illusions are exhausted.
>
> —*Arthur Miller*

The true use of the imagination is to decipher the present under its teeming incoherency and the anomalies of language…. As for the Future, your task is not to foresee, but to enable it. All true creation is not a prejudgment of the Future…but the apprehending of a new aspect of the present, which is a heap of raw materials bequeathed by the past…therefore let the future unfurl itself at leisure, like a tree putting forth its branches one by one.

—*Antoine de Saint-Exupery*

> Life never presents us with anything which may not be looked upon
> as a fresh starting point, no less than as a termination.
>
> —*André Gide*

> Fear not that life shall come to an end
> but rather that it shall never have a beginning.
>
> —*John Henry Cardinal Newman*

Crossing a threshold to a new life, especially one not chosen, is almost always jagged. In the context we are discussing—illness, addiction, and other trauma—it is almost always very painful, a moment, or a lifetime, where everything seems stripped away and your moorings are lost. The familiar is gone—taken—and in its place marches what seems like an eternal stream of chaos. The only real danger is that you stop in the middle, allowing the chaos to become frozen in time, creating its own endless stream of horror, allowing the past to dictate the present.

As you cross your threshold, as your life changes and transitions, there are also many opportunities. You are off on what hopefully can become the journey of a lifetime. Be prepared. Put on your seat belt, for the path might surprise you, shock you, anger you, delight you, comfort you, or even raise your level of consciousness, commitment, and appreciation for life. The quotations in *Words That Heal* may trigger some of these feelings and experiences. What is unlikely is that these words by some of our greatest sages and wisdom keepers, these sound bytes for the soul, will leave you unaffected or untouched.

So begins our journey of healing and recovery from life's disappointments. Remember that this new journey has invariably and necessarily started after an ending. Perhaps it is the end of a hope we had for our loved one, an end to a dream, or an opportunity for something more. We have lost something precious because of some kind of illness, addiction, or trauma. Something has been taken, and we must rise like the mythical phoenix or fall to depths of unimaginable despair and disenchantment.

Interestingly, the Chinese symbol for crisis is composed of two characters: danger and opportunity, which reminds us that a crisis is always the juncture between danger and opportunity. The stakes have never been higher to cross the threshold. The danger is present and real. Yet, we are also perched on a precipice that could lead us to levels of greater consciousness, appreciation, compassion, and love.

But before we can grasp the opportunities that chaos can hold for us, we must first understand the nature of the problem that stands in our way. When we do, we will find that there is no such thing as *the problem*, but rather *the problems*. Problems typically happen in bunches, often big bunches. This means that many times illness, addiction, and other traumas occur together within the same family. Today, many of our families face this triple threat.

What follows in the next chapter is a broad-ranging and encompassing statement of the problems we face, accompanied by snippets of specific dilemmas that address what is wrong and what we are up against as we face our troubles. We now live in severe times, times that call forth our greatest capacities for what may be the greatest possibility of all, human consciousness and survivorship, rather than unconsciousness and victimization.

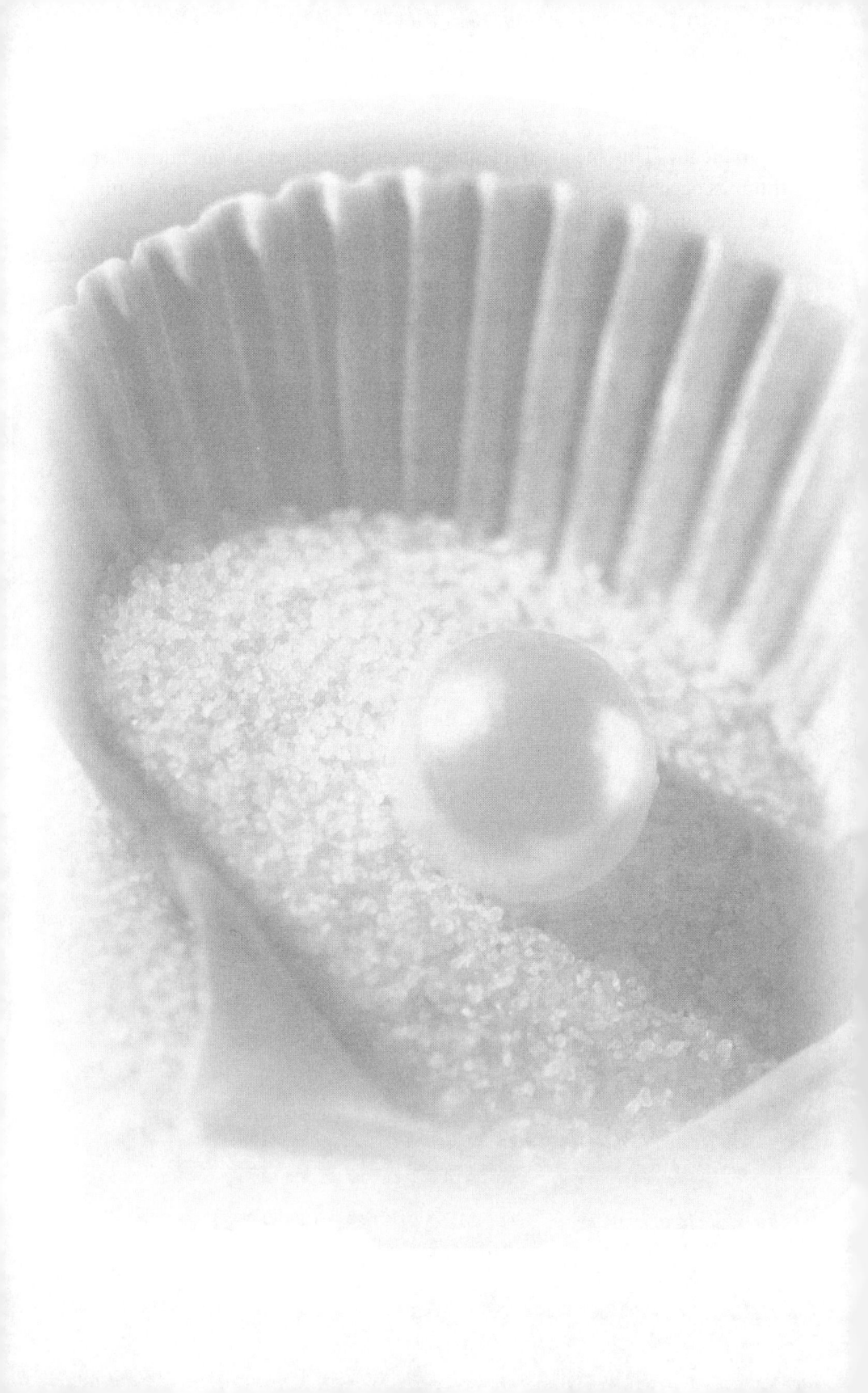

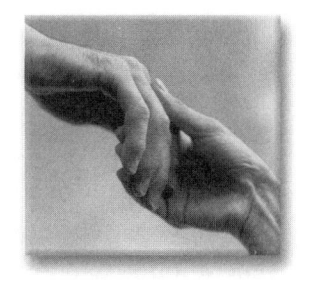

CHAPTER 2

The Problem

"Life is difficult," begins the very first paragraph of the twentieth-century classic, *The Road Less Travelled,* by M. Scott Peck. Few of us are able to avoid life's difficulties, much less life's tragedies, which seem to come in infinite varieties. Whether small or large, they always hurt. They always occasion pain. Yet, as wisdom keeper Benjamin Franklin reminds us, "What hurts, instructs." German philosopher Friedrich Nietzsche amplifies the point, "That which does not kill us makes us stronger."

Some of us wrestle with major *life circumstances*: poverty of mind, body, or soul; loss of family; abandonment; abuse, whether physical, sexual, or spiritual; and a host of other difficult as well as demanding assaults. Others wrestle with major *physical illnesses,* such as cancer, Parkinson's disease, Alzheimer's, traumatic brain injuries, chronic fatigue immune dysfunction syndrome, AIDS, fibromyalgia, multiple sclerosis, or environmental illness. Still others deal with *mental illnesses*, such as schizophrenia, bipolar disorder, major depression, or obsessive-compulsive disorder, all of which involve brain dysfunctions. In addition, many deal with life-threatening *addictions* including alcoholism and other drug dependencies as well as addictions to other substances, things (such as compulsive spending or shopping), and even people (such as sexual addiction). The numbers of us who are direct sufferers are staggering.

What is more, many believe that we live in what may be the most tumultuous time in all of history. As if the illnesses, addictions, and other traumas we encounter are not enough to experience and witness, our generation is exposed to an unprecedented explosion of information. We face more new information in a single day than previous generations were exposed to in a lifetime. In fact, much of what we learn today will be obsolete by tomorrow. We now change careers at least a dozen times over the course of our lives. We spend the equivalent of five days a year just opening and reading junk mail. We spend two hours or more each day commuting to and from our place of work.

In an age when we can have virtually all of the world's information in the palm of our hand, we also live in a world when our institutions are challenged as never before. One of our most sacred institutions, the church, has been rocked with scandal and outrage by the discovery that many clergy have abused our children. Moreover, for the first time, adults are afraid of children. In no other time in history have so many children murdered other children and adults. Much of this trauma occurs in another of our most sacred institutions, the school. Schoolyard shootings no longer grab the headlines because they are so common.

We are exposed to more violence than ever before, if only because we get to see it daily on television or read about it in newspapers, magazines, and periodicals. Almost every man, woman, and child, for example, has witnessed repeatedly the violent destruction of the Twin Towers of the World Trade Center, the symbol of America's financial strength, as well as the destruction of the Pentagon, a symbol of America's physical and intellectual strength. And as modern research in traumatic stress and traumatic grief shows, it often matters little whether we are the direct recipients of such adversity or are front-row witnesses.

Never before have the aftershocks of one day of infamy, 9/11, so changed our entire world. We now live with war, terrorism, and fear of homeland destruction as never before.

Chapter 2: The Problem

Never before have so many men and women been confused about what roles and what rules govern their lives. Who does what, when, how, and to whom are no longer universally agreed upon behaviors.

Never before has the planet been so small—and so troubled. Even the ozone layer that protects our planet is being pierced, the rain forests destroyed, and thousands of life forms are becoming extinct each year.

Our reactions to the problems presented by these horrors of all kinds are remarkably similar, and it matters little how we are exposed, whether directly or indirectly. The price remains enormous. Regardless of the size or shape, our problems seem to fill whatever space they occupy—or, as we will discover soon, whatever space we allow.

So it matters little whether you are good or bad, rich or poor, attractive or unattractive, intelligent or not. There are no exceptions to the journey of encountering problems—there is only preparation, fortitude, courage, strength, persistence, love, faith, hope, and, ultimately, triumph and healing.

> To be human is a problem.
>
> —*Abraham Heschel*

> We all suffer. Pain and sorrow find a niche in every household. All of us have lost people we loved. We have been betrayed or abandoned. We have made serious mistakes and have needed to forgive ourselves.
>
> —*Mary Pipher*

> Just about everybody is related to someone who is suffering from some form of illness, addiction, or other trauma.
>
> —*Herb Gravitz*

One in every five Americans experiences a mental disorder in any given year, and half of all Americans have such disorders at some time in their lives...mental illness, including suicide, is the second leading cause of disability after heart disease.... [But] nearly two-thirds of all people with diagnosable mental disorders do not seek treatment.... Treatment of mental disorders cost $69 billion in 1996...the nation spent $17.7 billion on Alzheimer's disease and $12.6 billion on treatment for drug and alcohol abuse that year. The figures do not include indirect costs, like days of work lost because of mental illness.

—David Satcher

Millions of kids now seek solace in machines.
We're losing them, like phantom children,
as they wrap their psyches around, and try to find comfort in,
the phosphorescent glow of the computer screen.

—Susan Skog

The National Institutes of Health recently released a study showing that 70 percent of all disease is stress related, and the World Health Organization warns of an increasing incidence of stress-related depression.

—Elaine St. James

If a person breaks a leg in the street, civil help tends to him quickly —ambulance, doctors, police. Break your mind and you lie there. The American community finds money for taking care of tens of millions —the poor, the aged, the physically ill. Why are there so many mentally ill people cut off from help?

—A.M. Rosenthal

> Epidemiologists find that at any given time,
> 75 percent of all people are "symptomatic,"
> experiencing physical or psychological distress.
> Yet most don't seek treatment,
> instead defining their distress as part of normal life.
>
> —*Froma Walsh*

Internationally, nearly 500 million people suffer from some type of mental illness, ranging from mild depression to chronic schizophrenia to substance abuse. Comprising half of the ten leading causes of disability, these illnesses account for 11 percent of incapacity in the world.

—*Rosalynn Carter*

> Approximately one-third of the single adult homeless
> population suffer from a severe mental illness,
> frequently co-occurring with alcohol and drug abuse.
>
> —*1992 Federal Task Force on Homelessness and Mental Illness*

Particularly within the past decade, there have been significant developments in professional practice with families. These include increasing evidence for the role of biological factors in serious mental illness.... Documentation of the devastating impact of mental illness on families.... Greater recognition of family contributions and expertise regarding their relative's treatment and recovery.

—*Diane Marsh*

> Unrecognized mental disorders
> account for 30 to 80 percent of all cases
> that primary-care physicians see in their offices.
>
> —Mental Health Policy Resource Center in Washington, D.C.

> Taking the most conservative statistical approach …
> over 100 million Americans have mental illness
> in their immediate families.
> And that's without counting extended kin and partners.
>
> —Victoria Secunda

In part, because of the stigma associated with it, the true impact of mental illness on our society and even the world is often nearly invisible. A landmark 1990 assessment of the global burden of disease by the Harvard School of Public Health, the World Health Organization, and the World Bank found that of the ten leading causes of disability (when measured in years lived with disability) in the world, half were psychiatric conditions—depression, alcohol use, manic depression, schizophrenia, and obsessive-compulsive disorder. It also determined that by the year 2020, the leading cause of disability in the world will be major depression.

—Rosalynn Carter

Pain is now detached from any context that could give it meaning and turned into a technical problem that has to be solved by the physician … in traditional cultures pain was a part of man's participation in a marred universe. Its meaning was cosmic and mythic and not individual and technical.

—Ivan Illich

> Alcoholism and alcohol abuse are associated with
> more violence, car accidents, boating accidents,
> childhood abuse, physical battering, suicide, and illness
> than virtually any other problem.
>
> —*National Association for Children of Alcoholics*

> Alcoholic treatment centers throughout the country
> report that over half of their patients are addicted to
> both alcohol and one or more prescription drugs.
>
> —*James Milam and Katherine Ketcham*

The fact is that the effects of alcohol simply cannot be generalized for both alcoholics and nonalcoholics. For most drinkers, alcohol is not addictive; but for the minority who are alcoholics, the criteria of true drug addiction are fulfilled: an increased tissue tolerance to the drug, a physical dependence on the drug with physical withdrawal symptoms, and an irresistible need for the drug when it is withdrawn.... Psychological symptoms are secondary to the physiological disease and not relevant to its onset.

—*James Milam and Katherine Ketcham*

> Recent estimates indicate there are between
> 28 and 34 million children of alcoholics,
> over half of them adults.
>
> —*National Association for Children of Alcoholics*

The accumulated evidence from all the life sciences positively indicates that physiology, not psychology, determines whether a drinker will become addicted to alcohol or not. The alcoholic's genes, enzymes, hormones, brain and other body chemistries work together to create his abnormal and unfortunate reaction to alcohol.

—Mel Schulstad

Those people who have both a mental illness
and a serious problem with drugs or alcohol
have far more than twice the difficulties
of people who have either one alone.

—Rebecca Woolis

We prefer to talk about our children's "hyperactivity" or "learning disability," rather than examine the inadequacy of our schools; we prefer to be told we suffer from "hypertension" rather than change our overcompetitive business world; we accept ever-increasing rates of cancer rather than investigate how the chemical industry poisons our goods to increase profits.

—Fritjof Capra

I feel like I am wearing a scarlet A,
only this stigma is because I suffer from mental illness.

—Primary sufferer of the mental illness schizophrenia

In a society that claims to support "family values,"
most families have instead been viewed through a glass darkly;
their strengths and potential have gone unseen and undervalued.

—Froma Walsh

Chapter 2: The Problem

In an age when we face an average of twenty-three adversities a day, most of us are ill-equipped to manage, let alone thrive, amid such unprecedented demands.... *USA Today* reports that in a typical day office workers send and receive 163 messages via phone, fax, e-mail, interoffice mail, and cell phone. That number doubles every year.

—Elaine St. James

So many people walk around with a meaningless life.
They seem half-asleep,
even when they are busy doing things they think are important.
This is because they're chasing the wrong things.

—Morrie Schwartz

In our collective denial, we have turned health into a personal responsibility rather than a social concern; we diagnose many of our difficulties coping with a sick society and a toxic environment as individual health problems.

—Kat Duff

The interminably ill are still a largely unidentified segment of the population. Estimates have it that nearly forty-three million people in the United States have cardiovascular disease, ten or eleven million have diabetes, more that one-half million have lupus, and about 250,000 have multiple sclerosis. Add to the list severe asthma, arthritis, hemophilia, a variety of liver, kidney, and intestinal disorders, endometriosis, physiologically based mental illness, and others yet to be diagnosed and named, and it becomes apparent that people with degenerative and intermittently life-threatening illnesses hardly form an exclusive society.

—Cheri Register

Mental illness makes you feel devoid of meaning;
it makes you feel devoid of hope.
And the loss of hope is one of the most tremendous losses
for people who suffer mental illness.

—*Rosalynn Carter*

It is too easy to blame the fragility of American families on the failure of individuals to acquire the "right" values. The bigger problem is that families have been abandoned by society to solve, on their own, the increasingly complex problems of their individual members. In applying a version of rugged individualism to the family, we have increasingly isolated an institution whose health requires the nourishment of public, social, and legislative support.

—*David A. Karp*

Life doesn't meet you halfway;
you have to meet life all the way.

—*Gurudev (Yogi Amrit Desai)*

Our culture breeds intolerance for personal suffering; we avert our gaze from disability, avoid contact with the bereaved, and dispense chirpy advice to "cheer up" and get over catastrophic events.

—*Froma Walsh*

Our culture is at war with families.

—*Mary Pipher*

> Pain and suffering are not exceptions to the human condition;
> they are inevitable players in the drama of our lives.
>
> —Rev. Wayne Muller

> I was always going so fast…
> until I finally figured out I wasn't getting anywhere.
>
> —Family member

> Where is God when you need him?
>
> —C. S. Lewis

Family members feel great ambivalence in messages that offer confusion about obligations to self and others, devalue caring work (teaching and caregiving), privatize family life, and increasingly withdraw structural support from a system already dramatically overloaded with obligations. The government is indifferent to its needs. The fate of American families must be viewed as a national problem, and, as such, it is the responsibility of federal and state governments to intervene in revitalizing troubled families. The fates of societies and families are intertwined. Societies must care for and nourish families in order to ensure members can extend compassionate care to each other during moments of vulnerability, crisis, and illness.

—David A. Karp

> Social isolation is just as dangerous as smoking.
>
> —Mary Pipher

A shame-based person will guard against exposing his inner self to others, but more significantly, he will guard against exposing himself to himself. Toxic shame is so excruciating because it is the painful exposure of the believed failure of self to self. In toxic shame the self becomes an object that can't be trusted. As an object that can't be trusted, one experiences oneself as untrustworthy.

—*John Bradshaw*

We begin life with loss.
We are cast from the womb without an apartment,
a charge plate, a job, or a car.
We are sucking, sobbing, clinging, helpless babies.

—*Judith Viorst*

The complete absence of fear
suggests some kind of brain damage.

—*Parent of a child with OCD*

Illness is the night-side of life, a more onerous citizenship. Everyone who is born holds dual citizenship, in the kingdom of the well and in the kingdom of the sick. Although we all prefer to use only the good passport, sooner or later each of us is obliged, at least for a spell, to identify ourselves as citizens of that other place.

—*Susan Sontag*

Prejudice is the reason of fools.

—*Voltaire*

> To dare is to lose one's footing momentarily.
> To not dare is to lose oneself.
>
> —*Soren Kierkegaard*

> Modern medicine has helped lengthen the life span,
> giving rise to the need for transgenerational caretaking.
>
> —*Florence Kaslow*

> We neglect the positive value of affection….
> Today the world is very complicated,
> and much suffering has happened
> due to lack of human sympathy and human affection.
>
> —*Dalai Lama*

It should be no surprise to any of us that heart disease is the leading killer in our country. No shock that depression is epidemic. Our physical health increasingly reflects the pain we share on a spiritual level. I believe our hearts and spirits literally ache from denying our humanity. They weep at how disconnected we've become from one another and from the earth. They mourn the absence of compassion throughout much of our culture.

—*Susan Skog*

> Those who desire to give up freedom in order to gain security
> will not have, nor will they deserve, either.
>
> —*Thomas Jefferson*

You will find that my bed exactly fits you,
whether you are short or tall!

—*Procrustes*

None but a coward dares to boast
that he has never known fear.

—*Marshal Ferdinand Foch*

It is what we think we know already
that often prevents us from learning.

—*Claude Bernard*

One must be thrust out of a finished cycle in life, and…part with one's faith, one's love, when one would rather renew the faith and recreate the passion. [There is no recreation, just creation!]

—*Anaïs Nin*

Everybody wants to be somebody; nobody wants to grow.

—*Goethe*

The road to mental hell is paved with gossip.

—*Robert and Jane Alter*

The world fears a new experience more than it fears anything. Because a new experience displaces so many old experiences… the world doesn't fear a new idea. It can pigeonhole any idea. But it can't pigeonhole a real new experience.

—D. H. Lawrence

Our deepest fear is not that we are inadequate. Our deepest fear is that we are powerful beyond measure. It is our light that most frightens us. We ask ourselves, "Who am I to be brilliant, gorgeous, talented, fabulous?" Actually, who are you not to be? You are a child of God. Your playing small does not serve the world. There's nothing enlightened about shrinking so that other people won't feel insecure around you. We are all meant to shine as children do. We were born to make manifest the glory of God that is within us. It's not just in some of us; it's in everyone. And as we let our own light shine, we unconsciously give other people permission to do the same. As we're liberated from our own fear, our presence automatically liberates others.

—Marianne Williamson

Studies show that early childhood losses make us sensitive to losses we encounter later on. And so, in mid-life, our response to a death in the family, a divorce, the loss of a job, may be a severe depression—the response of that helpless and hopeless, and angry, child.

—Judith Viorst

Insanity is doing the same thing over and over again, but expecting different results.

—Rita Mae Brown

There is often less danger in the things we fear
than the things we desire.

—*John Hollen*

Well, for one thing, the culture we have does not make people feel good about themselves. We're teaching the wrong things. And you have to be strong enough to say if the culture doesn't work, don't buy it. Create your own. Most people can't do it. They're more unhappy than me—even in my current condition. [He was dying of ALS when he said this.]

—*Morrie Schwartz*

It is not because things are difficult that we do not dare;
it is because we do not dare that they are difficult.

—*Seneca*

You have made me a keeper of vineyards,
yet my own vineyard I have not kept.

—*Song of Solomon*

When you point your finger in blame,
there are three pointing back at you.

—*Anonymous*

Argue for your limitations, and sure enough, they're yours.

—*Richard Bach*

Chapter 2: The Problem

We do not see things as they are.
We see them as we are.

—Talmud

What lies beyond us and what lies before us are tiny matters
when compared to what lies within us.

—Ralph Waldo Emerson

To repel one's cross is to make it heavier.

—Henri Frederic Amiel

All of the facts belong only to the problem,
not its solution.

—Ludwig Wittgenstein

Life is not so much a problem to be solved
as a mystery to be lived.

—Anonymous

The wave is ignorant of the true nature of the sea:
how can the temporal comprehend the eternal?

—Sa'ib of Tabriz

'Tis better to have loved and lost
than never to have loved at all.

—*Alfred Lord Tennyson*

Most of us do not today believe
that whatever the ups and downs of detail
within our limited experience,
the larger whole is primarily beautiful.

—*Gregory Bateson*

We do not err because truth is difficult to see.
It is visible at a glance.
We err because this is more comfortable.

—*Alexander Solzhenitsyn*

You can outdistance that which is running after you,
but you cannot outdistance that which is running inside you.

—*African proverb*

Ultimately we know deeply
that the other side of every fear is a freedom.

—*Marilyn Ferguson*

We must accept finite disappointment,
but we must never lose infinite hope.

—*Martin Luther King, Jr.*

Chapter 2: The Problem

Hope is necessary in every condition.
The miseries of poverty, sickness, of captivity, would,
without this comfort, be insupportable.

—*Samuel Johnson*

Gray skies are just clouds passing over.

—*Duke Ellington*

We are all in the gutter, but some of us are looking at the stars.

—*Oscar Wilde*

A pessimist is someone
who complains about the noise
when opportunity knocks.

—*Michael Levine*

Optimism is making the most of all that comes
and the least of all that goes.

—*Anonymous*

When pessimists think they're taking a chance,
optimists feel they're grasping a great opportunity.

—*Anonymous*

Our greatest weakness lies in giving up.
The most certain way to succeed
is always to try just one more time.

—*Thomas Edison*

Contrary to popular belief, it is not so much fear of denial
as it is confusion and embarrassment
that keep people out of the doctor's office
in the early stages of illness.

—*Cheri Register*

If you can't voice the pain,
you can't feel the emotions.

—*Family member*

There is no object so foul
that intense light will not make it beautiful.

—*Ralph Waldo Emerson*

I will never ever forget that call. It was 8 A.M. The voice at the other end of the phone asked to speak to Mr. or Mrs. Smith. In a rather cold and detached way, the person said this was the university hospital. Our son was admitted an hour ago because he was running through the dorms naked and shouting obscenities. We knew he could be different from others—he really always was—but this—this was just too much. It began a nightmare that hasn't ended to this day.

—*Distraught parent*

Chapter 2: The Problem

> Powerlessness corrupts.
>
> —*Michael Lerner*

―᙮―

> No one understands—and I have given up trying.
>
> —*Family member*

―᙮―

When the family can be characterized as traumatized, then the family environment can be characterized as burned out.... The environment of a traumatized family is ultimately sterile. Whether the family members are disengaged or engaged in conflict, are inexpressive or express affection, are depressed or lead busy productive lives, there is still something missing in the home environment. That something is the spontaneous, authentic, real essence of each family member. Each member is less than full there. Significant aspects of each family member's full range of emotions, thoughts, and needs are missing. The result is that family members do not really feel connected with one another. They do not know each other in the complete manner that is possible for people whose lives are intimately connected.

> —*Charles R. Figley*

―᙮―

> Absence makes the heart grow frozen, not fonder.
>
> —*Judith Viorst*

―᙮―

Passionate investment leaves us vulnerable to loss. And sometimes, no matter how clever we are, we must lose.... For the road to human development is paved with renunciation. Throughout our life we grow by giving up.

> —*Judith Viorst*

―᙮―

The family is now seen as a form of cultural "foreplay," preparing the individual for intercourse with the real world. The family is viewed as little more than a temporary training ground, to be used and even abused until the nest becomes empty or a parent "gives away" their child to someone else in a marital ceremony that speaks of forsaking all others while the respective families of the new marital partners sit divided on opposite sides of the church and temple.

—Paul Pearsall

As if in a trance, addicted people set aside their alleged values and sometimes ruthlessly pursue their addiction.

—Charlotte Davis Kasl

After twenty years,
hospice still provides care to a minority
of dying persons in the United States.

—William Lamers, Jr.

Whereas loss is an occasion for family and community cohesion in most cultures, Americans worry about "intruding" on the grief of others and are wary about facing their own mortality and loss.

—Froma Walsh

Often I am not where I am,
but where my thoughts lead me.

—Thomas à Kempis

One thing that comes out in myths is that at the bottom of the abyss comes the voice of salvation. The black moment is the moment when the real message of transformation is going to come. At the darkest moment comes the light.

—Joseph Campbell

If you are distressed by anything external,
the pain is not due to the thing itself
but to your own estimate of it.
This you have the power to revise at any moment.

—Marcus Aurelius

We are all the products
of thousands of years of failed parenting…
because the human species has not yet evolved to the point
that it knows how to raise its young without injury.

—Harville Hendrix

Violence is the real sex now.

—Mary Pipher

Mystics and schizophrenics find themselves in the same ocean,
but the mystics swim whereas the schizophrenics drown.

—R. D. Laing

If we are to achieve a richer culture...we must recognize the whole gamut of human potentialities, and so weave a less arbitrary social fabric, one in which each diverse human gift will find a fitting place.

—*Margaret Mead*

Life is a contest of opposites: birth and death; health and sickness; love and hate; giving and taking; systole and diastole; summer and winter; day and night.

—*E. A. Bennett*

Fear always springs from ignorance.

—*Ralph Waldo Emerson*

It is only because of problems that we grow mentally and spiritually...when we avoid the legitimate suffering that results from dealing with problems, we also avoid the growth that problems demand from us.

—*M. Scott Peck*

When we speak to God we are said to be praying, but when God speaks to us we are said to be schizophrenic.

—*Lily Tomlin*

The family is generally not a sick place. The family is suffering from severe neglect.

—*Paul Pearsall*

Western culture emphasizes personal responsibility, in the belief that we are masters of our own fate. In U.S. society, we hold a curious split image of individual and family responsibility, crediting individuals for their success but blaming their families for any failures.

—*Froma Walsh*

The question is not whether we will die,
but how we will live.

—*Joan Borysenko*

We have found the enemy, and it is us.

—*Pogo Possum*

One of the ways in which people have tried to make sense of the world's suffering in every generation has been by assuming that we deserve what we get, that somehow our misfortunes come as punishment for our sins.

—*Rabbi Harold S. Kushner*

Not that I am (I think) in much danger of ceasing to believe in God. The real danger is of coming to believe such dreadful things about Him. The conclusion I dread is not, "So there's no God after all," but, "So this is what God's really like. Deceive yourself no longer."

—*C. S. Lewis*

A man who goes to a psychiatrist should have his head examined.

—*Sam Goldwyn*

What surprises you most about mankind? They lose their health to make money and then lose their money to restore their health. By thinking anxiously about the future, they forget the present, such that they live neither for the present nor for the future and they live as if they will never die, and they die as if they never lived.

—*Confucius*

Indeed, nothing has caused more problems for our species, created more pain, produced more suffering, or resulted in more tragedy, than that which was intended to bring us our greatest joy—our relationships with each other.

—*Neale Donald Walsch*

We fear our highest possibilities (as well as our lowest ones). We are generally afraid to become that which we can glimpse in our most perfect moments, under the most perfect conditions, under conditions of greatest courage. We enjoy and even thrill to the Godlike possibilities we see in ourselves in such peak moments. And yet we simultaneously shiver with weakness, awe, and fear before these very same possibilities.

—*Abraham Maslow*

If you set out to be less than you are capable of being,
I warn you,
you will be deeply unhappy for the rest of your life.

—*Abraham Maslow*

Chapter 2: The Problem

> Problems call forth our courage and our wisdom;
> indeed they create our courage and wisdom.
> It is only because of problems
> that we grow mentally and spiritually.
>
> —*M. Scott Peck*

―∞―

The serious problems in life…are never fully resolved. If ever they should appear to be so it is a sure sign that something has been lost. The meaning and purpose of a problem seems to lie not in its solution but in our working at it incessantly.

—*Carl Jung*

―∞―

It takes little to document the immense problems that we face in today's technological world. They come from all sides—from within the body and from without. As we have seen, they are biological, political, technological, psychological, spiritual, even philosophical. There is little question that as a country, and as a community of countries, we are undergoing enormous changes that have a profound effect on all families everywhere. Families need more support, not less.

A major article written by Dr. Florence W. Kaslow, one of the founders of family therapy, in the *American Psychologist*, perhaps the most prestigious of all psychological professional journals, discusses these challenging changes. She writes: "As the new century begins to unfold, families in virtually every country are experiencing great turbulence and living in tumultuous circumstances…. At the microsystemic level (individual and personal realms of living), families reflect the problems of the larger contexts in which they live. Many are plagued by stresses caused by radical changes in the economic and sociopolitical spheres of their society, which resulted from either social revolution or war."

The above statements are not meant to deny the realities of biological or biochemical causes of problems such as serious mental illness, but rather to put them in the greater social context. Illness and social ills can never be separated from the broader social context, because they are dependent upon cultural norms, interpretations, and social values. Government responses reflect social stereotypes and prejudices, and reveal that attitudes toward illness and social problems have strong ideological and moral components. For example, what merits "reimbursement" under health insurance is as much a socio-political decision as a medical decision.

Regardless of governmental and societal influence, the great American humorist Mark Twain reminds us, "Life is one damn thing after another, but trouble is the same damn thing again and again." Many problems are minor and are the fuel for our "growing pains." Some, however, lead to bigger issues and actually need to be more fully understood before we can act properly and utilize the opportunities that they afford as fuel for the journey.

We need a closer look at what we are up against. We need to have a way to name these obstacles and to find a way to create them as openings to a new future. A predominant and significant theme throughout the words of all of the great thinkers is that life's losses and difficulties—whatever their causes—are opportunities and doorways to growth and wisdom.

It is to this task of naming our problems that we now turn, for the beginning of wisdom is to call things by their right name. It is an invaluable step on the road to healing and to triumph. It is the foundation upon which the odyssey is built. A popular bumper sticker says, "If we don't know where we are headed, it's not likely we'll get there." The art of diagnosis, which is one way of naming our problems, is the art of discovery, for diagnosis opens the door to learning something important about yourself and, perhaps, someone you love. While a diagnosis closes some doors, it opens others; while a diagnosis doesn't end life, it does redirect it.

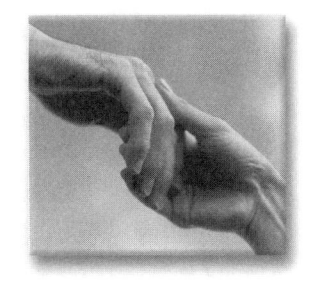

CHAPTER 3

The Diagnoses

All effective understanding begins with an accurate assessment and analysis of the problem. We have recently discovered that it is also imperative to assess the impact of the problem on those it touches, which most often is the family. One way to accomplish these tasks is to assign a name, or a label, to the problem. Names can be formal, such as the diagnostic labels of illnesses that insurance companies will pay for. They can also be more informal—names such as fear, grief, loss—ones that insurance companies will not pay for.

While diagnosis and assessment are similar terms, even confused for each other at times, there are important differences. A diagnosis tends to be a more stable and inclusive summation of the core problem, while an assessment is the consideration of the moment-to-moment responses and their impact that an individual makes to a situation. An assessment is much more specific, temporary, and easy to describe. Like a more formal diagnosis, assessment can facilitate healing and recovery by helping to understand the problem.

There are advantages and disadvantages of labels or other ways that are used to formulate diagnoses. At their best, diagnoses point to effective treatment protocols and help explain confusing and contradictory behaviors. Without the compass of a good working diagnosis or clinical assessment, no one—not the doctor, not the patient, not the family—knows what the problems really are. Turmoil reigns as the increasing stress, loss, grief, and exhaustion continue. The result is a corresponding loss of the possibilities and options that are also present in the rubble.

One parent expressed the positive aspect of a diagnosis in the following way: "If we didn't know that our son's erratic behavior stemmed from a biochemical disorder, we'd be lost in some deep, dark, and scary forest with no way out. At least now, we can see a path and have some direction." In this case, an accurate diagnosis opened the door to a set of new beliefs, each with different possibilities that the parents may have never seen in its absence.

Until an accurate diagnosis or assessment of the problem is formulated, there is almost always chaos and confusion. Undetected and unrecognized, illness, addiction, and trauma become the foreground, or main stage, upon which family life is enacted and the primary matrix or context in which the family interacts. Only with proper attention and recognition can these problems move into the background of the family experience where they belong.

One family member compared having a diagnosis to swimming in a fish pond: "The diagnosis lets you know what kind of water you're in," he said. He explained: "There are all kinds of diagnoses, just like there are all kinds of ponds. Some ponds are warm and friendly. They have beautiful flora. Non-aggressive fish swim there. Others are cold, dark, and murky." He continued: "With one type of diagnosis, one that is socially acceptable, you may be swimming in warm and clear water. There is little turbulence. Life flows. You even can get support. But if you have another diagnosis, like you are mentally ill, or even if you have cancer, then you're thrown into a cold, dreary, and scary place where there are fish [for example, doctors, nurses, hospitals, insurance companies, even the police at times] that you've never met before—and they are often not friendly! They can bite, they can be mean, and some of them can be downright nasty."

Diagnosis at its best is like an X-ray of the structure of the problem. It reveals the essence of the issues and points to directions for treatment.

For example, a diagnosis of cancer is predicated on the basis of the presence of a tumor; the diagnosis of Parkinson's points to a disturbance in the nervous system; the diagnosis of alcoholism shows the presence of problems in major areas of life that are associated with drinking; the diagnosis of psychosis reveals a break in the perception of reality; the diagnosis of obsessive-compulsive disorder affirms the presence of obsessions and compulsions; and the diagnosis of bipolar disorder attests to a disturbance of high and low moods.

Often, diagnoses come suddenly, even unexpectedly. If the fish pond metaphor is expanded, a diagnosis can be the equivalent of swimming in a familiar pond and then being picked up by the collar and dumped into another one that is cold, dark, and murky. There is no welcome sign or mat to guide you around the dangerous rocks and crevices.

When a diagnosis is used respectfully, the way it is intended, then light can be shed where there was darkness. However, all diagnoses have pluses and minuses. At their worst, diagnoses stigmatize, marginalize, polarize, and otherwise isolate and separate the ill from the broader system. It matters little who you are as a person; you are seen as an illness, addiction, or other trauma. While it is true, too, that a diagnosis can be unreliable and does not take into account the unique differences and strengths of the individual or family, it can be important to have some idea of where we are to begin and where we are going. It is critical to have a sense of the terrain in which our encounter will unfold.

What diagnoses rarely show, however, are the "side effects" of the particular problem—what I have called "core issues" in some of my previous writings. These side effects include negative symptoms such as depression, guilt, low self-esteem, confusion, denial, low motivation, apathy, and often a loss of self. These issues typically accompany any illness, addiction, or other trauma and affect every member of the family, even though they are not always addressed. They can affect the "primary sufferer," the one directly experiencing the problem, or the "secondary sufferer," or the family, loved ones, friends, and even associates of the person with the problem.

Despite its limitations, a diagnosis is often the starting point of effective help. It is important to understand that there may be different diagnoses for different family members. While they experience circumstances differently and are not equally affected, virtually all loved ones are impacted. And the lack of a formal diagnosis does not mean there are not problems that block or retard movement forward. Living under the influence of illness, addiction, or other trauma casts a very long shadow.

The official manual of diagnosis and classification of mental disorders (by the American Psychiatric Association) is known simply as the *Diagnostic and Statistical Manual of Mental Disorders*. It is currently in its fourth revision and is called *DSM-IV* for short. Contrary to *DSM-IV*, most emotional distress and behavioral disturbances are not mental illnesses. True mental illnesses are medical conditions caused by chemical and structural imbalances and abnormalities in the brain that interfere with a person's ability to function effectively. They include obsessive-compulsive disorder, schizophrenia, bipolar disorder, and autism. They do not include most of the anxiety states, most depressions, and most behaviors that are displeasing or upsetting to others. No medical tests exist yet to diagnose mental illness.

Do not be deterred by the "technical" nature of some diagnoses. And even though you may find a diagnosis demeaning, pejorative, or stigmatizing, you will still most likely have to deal with it. The professionals with whom you may have to interact will use these terms. It is your responsibility to know the playing court that you enter into. Learn the vocabulary because you will be required to understand and to speak the language. You will find that it will be much easier to navigate the system—or fish tank—when you can understand and use the language correctly.

Chapter 3: The Diagnoses

As long as an enemy is invisible,
it is invincible.

—*Richard Dannelley*

No problem can be solved
from the same consciousness that created it.
We must learn to see the world anew.

—*Albert Einstein*

Effective treatment begins
with an accurate diagnosis carefully conceived.

—*Herb Gravitz*

Discovery consists of looking at the same thing as everyone else and
perceiving something different.

—*Albert Szent-Gyorgyi*

Of all the knowledge,
the wise and good seek most to know themselves.

—*William Shakespeare*

A diagnosis is like the defroster on your car.
It can't change the weather out there,
but it can let you see what you're dealing with.

—*Family member*

A diagnosis closes some doors, and it opens others.
—Herb Gravitz

You can't recover from what you do not understand.
—Lillian Hellman

The truth will set you free....
But first it will make you miserable.
—Nathaniel Branden

Never go to a doctor whose office plants have died.
—Erma Bombeck

There is no healthy way to adapt to alcoholism.
—Sharon Wegscheider

The essential feature of post-traumatic stress disorder [PTSD] is the development of characteristic symptoms following exposure to an extreme traumatic stressor involving direct personal experience of an event that involves actual or threatened death or serious injury, or other threat to one's physical integrity; *or witnessing an event* [emphasis added] that involves death, injury, or a threat to the physical integrity of another person; or learning about unexpected or violent death, serious harm, or threat of death or *injury experienced by a family member or other close associate* [emphasis added].

—DSM-IV

Chapter 3: The Diagnoses

In the beginning, my own intense denial of my illness, and how it would have an impact on my life in the years ahead, was accompanied by an explosive rage, welling up from deep within me. That rage eventually unleashed my strength, my courage, my ability to survive, and my passion to make a positive difference in the world. But first I had to acknowledge my anger fully to myself.

—*Linda Noble Topf*

The family illness we are studying is basically the same no matter what chemical is being abused— alcohol, prescription drugs, marijuana, cocaine, street drugs, whatever.

—*Sharon Wegscheider*

The effect on family life begins with the way a diagnosis is delivered. The doctors give a diagnosis, but they frequently don't translate what it will mean into psychosocial terms for the family.... The first five minutes of communication at the critical turning point of diagnosis can set up an emotional model for the whole course of the illness.... Who says what to whom matters a great deal. Whatever a doctor does at that vulnerable time can influence people for years.

—*John S. Rolland*

Not to know is bad, but not to wish to know is worse.

—*African proverb*

The meaning of the diagnosis to family members is important to determine. Some families perceive illness as a challenge, whereas other families see the same illness as punishment. Some diagnoses united families (everyone in our family has back pain), whereas other diagnoses initially estranged family members (e.g., mental illness, abuse, AIDS).... Families have taught us that *it is the belief about the problem that is the problem.* If a family is experiencing cancer, for example, it is its beliefs about the cancer—its origin, the likely outcome for the person and the family, what treatment to use—that create difficulties, not the cancer itself. Beliefs have a pivotal profound, and palpable influence on families' experiences with illness and other problems.

—*Drs. Wright, Watson, and Bell*

A questioning man is halfway to being wise.

—*Irish proverb*

Because scientists believe that severe and persistent mental illness is a brain disorder, mental illness and severe and persistent mental illness also mean the same as brain disorder....We are only now moving out of the darkness and into the light in understanding brain disorders. It is very hard to grasp this medical model of mental illness.

—*E. Farrell and J. Murphy*

Biology is not destiny.

—*Norman Cousins*

Schizophrenia is a disturbance that lasts for at least six months and includes at least one month of active-phase symptoms (i.e., two or more of the following: delusions, hallucinations, disorganized speech, grossly disorganized or catatonic behavior, negative symptoms).

—DSM-IV

An addict is a frustrated mystic.
—William James

The essential features of obsessive-compulsive disorder [OCD] are recurrent obsessions or compulsions (Criterion A) that are severe enough to be time consuming (i.e., they take more than one hour a day) or cause marked distress or significant impairment (Criterion C). At some point during the course of the disorder, the person has recognized that the obsessions or compulsions are excessive or unreasonable (Criterion B).

—DSM-IV

Bipolar I Disorder is characterized by
one or more Manic or Mixed Episodes,
usually accompanied by Major Depressive Episodes.

—DSM-IV

Bipolar II Disorder is characterized by one or more
Major Depressive Episodes accompanied by
a least one Hypomanic Episode.

—DSM-IV

Major Depressive Disorder is characterized by one or more Major Depressive Episodes (i.e., at least two weeks of depressed mood or loss of interest accompanied by at least four additional symptoms of depression).

—DSM-IV

Dysthymic Disorder is characterized by at least two years of depressed mood for more days than not, accompanied by additional depressive symptoms that do not meet criteria for a Major Depressive Episode.

—DSM-IV

A Personality Disorder is an enduring pattern of inner experience and behavior that deviates markedly from the expectations of the individual's culture, is pervasive and inflexible, has an onset in adolescence or early adulthood, is stable over time and leads to distress or impairment.

—DSM-IV

The narrowest definition of psychotic is restricted to delusions or prominent hallucinations with the hallucinations occurring in the absence of insight into their pathological nature. A slightly less restrictive definition would also include prominent hallucinations that the individual realizes are hallucinatory experiences. Broader still is a definition that also includes other positive symptoms of Schizophrenia (i.e., disorganized speech, grossly disorganized or catatonic behavior).

—DSM-IV

You cannot treat an inpatient on an outpatient basis.

—*Carol Primeau*

A dual diagnosis is one that is a combination
of mental illness and substance abuse.

—*Herb Gravitz*

When the person with the illness or disorder is replaced with the identity of the diagnosis, as when a person with a psychosis becomes simply a "psychotic," or a schizophrenic condition becomes simply "a schizophrenic," then a disservice is done to the person as well as the family.

—*Herb Gravitz*

Are you up to your destiny?

—*Hamlet*

Not all families with a chronically disturbed member are severely dysfunctional as a family unit. In fact, given the evidence for a biological component in schizophrenia, affective disorders, substance abuse, and most probably other severe and chronic mental disturbances, family pathology may be neither a necessary nor a sufficient factor for the development of major psychiatric disorders.

—*Froma Walsh and Carol Anderson*

The absence of alternatives clears the mind marvelously.

—*Henry Kissinger*

The anxiety disorders are the most common of all mental illnesses.

—*National Institute of Mental Health*

Within the next five years, scientists are predicting that we will have faster-acting, more effective medications with fewer side effects, drugs that are targeted more specifically to particular neurotransmitters and their receptors. Some researchers even speculate that in a decade or two, there will be medications that prevent mental illnesses from developing in the first place in people who are genetically vulnerable.

—*Rosalynn Carter*

The essential feature of post-traumatic disorder is the development of characteristic symptoms following exposure…*or witnessing an event* that involves death, injury, or a threat to the physical integrity of another person; or learning about unexpected or violent death, serious harm, or threat of death *or injury experienced by a family member or other close associates* [italics added].

—*Charles R. Figley*

Well, at least I know what has been dogging me this whole time!

—*Family member*

As hard as it was to hear our son had a serious illness, there was a lot of relief and, as strange as it may seem, even a feeling of satisfaction. Jan (his wife) and I knew something was wrong all along. We just didn't know what. For a long time we thought that maybe we were just imagining things or blowing them out of proportion. Then, you know, you can get used to almost anything. But we knew. It wasn't in our mind.

—*Father of a child with a neurobiological disorder*

Chapter 3: The Diagnoses

> Nothing is more punitive than to give a disease meaning—that meaning being invariably a moralistic one.
>
> —*Susan Sontag*

> The Americans with Disabilities Act of 1990 (ADA) mandates that businesses with fifteen employees or more cannot discriminate against a qualified job candidate or employee on the basis of disability and must make reasonable accommodations for employees who have a mental illness.
>
> —*American Disabilities Act of 1990*

> It is difficult to overestimate the power of receiving a medical diagnosis. Since diagnosis of mental illness remains deeply stigmatizing, it is not surprising the "patient" often rejects it.
>
> —*David A. Karp*

> In an odd sort of way, I felt good about being diagnosed as a manic-depressive. For one thing, I knew I was going to have some highs as well as just lows. I also knew that the manic depression is a biochemical disorder and I can take medicine. I know the side effects can be difficult, but at least I know I don't have a weak will. It kind of takes the pressure off. I am not a bad person; I just have an illness—and thank God there is treatment. I am pretty sure my dad had it, but he never got the help he needed. There was no lithium then.
>
> —*A man diagnosed with Bipolar II disorder*

> We're so fond of each other because our ailments are the same.
>
> —*Jonathan Swift*

> Everyone who is born holds dual citizenship
> in the kingdom of the well and the kingdom of the sick.
>
> —*Susan Sontag*

When the doctor told me I had cancer, I was stunned. I just went numb. What about my family? How would they get by? What about my wife? Hell, how would *I* get by? I don't want to die. I left the doctor's office and that's when it hit me. I just cried and cried.

—*Newly diagnosed man with testicular cancer*

A part of me felt a certain satisfaction. At least people will know that I really can't do everything like before. It's a symbol that there really is something wrong and there is a reason I can't do things. When people ask me why I can't take care of things the way I used to, I can tell them, "I have been diagnosed with lupus."

—*A woman newly diagnosed*

> Illness has too often become a personal failure
> rather than a breakdown of normal health.
>
> —*Herb Gravitz*

> Be willing to have it so acceptance of what has happened is the first
> step to overcoming the consequences of any misfortune.
>
> —*William James*

Whatever limitations there are that relate to diagnosing the person who has the disorder—that is, the primary patient or sufferer—a diagnosis will at least begin to address some of the boundaries and parameters of the problem. What is much more hidden, more secret, and even less discussed is the countless numbers of secondary sufferers, the family, loved ones, and friends of the primary patient. Their wounds have been barely noticed—except by them, of course.

What we also need in order to be helpful to every member of the family is a way of describing or "diagnosing" the wounds of those who care for the wounded. Then, and only then, will we be addressing all the members of the family. Without including them, the primary sufferer will not get the help he or she needs, because the family may be too stressed, traumatized, grieved, overwhelmed, exhausted, and isolated.

None of the following "diagnoses" that characterize the plight of the secondary sufferer appear in *DSM-IV*, or are they even hinted at in this "bible." They are nevertheless critical in our exploration of the wake of illness, addiction, and other trauma. The addition of these "secondary diagnoses" incurred by the "non-ill" family members completes the family assessment and family diagnosis.

The focus is now appropriately on the entire family—in fact, even the future generations of the family can become a focus of healing. I tell my clients that every major or important decision that they make regarding their loved one's should be funneled through the future, projected needs, and values of every family member. Whether an adult loved one is allowed to live at home or not work, for example, should be considered in the light of how this decision will affect everyone in the family not only now, but a month from now, six months from now, a year from now, five years and even ten or twenty or thirty years from now.

It is to these hitherto unmentioned—even hidden—diagnoses that we next turn. Those with these diagnoses, while generally not formal and explicit, are more often unrecognized. The plight of these sufferers is even more often denied and minimized. There is little sense of entitlement for their pain and wounds that they receive from others. They often feel cut off and disenfranchised from help. Often, they experience insult to their injury.

There is a cost to caring...
nearly all of the attention has been directed
to people in harm's way [i.e., the primary sufferer]
and little to those who care for and worry about them
[i.e., the secondary sufferer].

—Charles R. Figley

As little as we know of illness, we know even less of care.
As much as the ill person's experience is denied,
the caregiver's experience is denied more completely.

—Arthur Frank

I am the co-patient! Somebody please get this!

—Spouse of a man with a neurobiological disorder (NBD)

There is a fundamental difference between the sequelae or pattern of response during and following a traumatic event for those exposed to primary and secondary stressors. The fundamental difference is that the primary trauma victim experiences symptoms that are directly associated with some aspect of the traumatic event, whereas the secondary trauma victim experiences symptoms that are associated with the primary trauma victim.

—Charles R. Figley

But what about us. No one is taking us seriously.

—Frustrated spouse

Chapter 3: The Diagnoses

> No one understands me.
> I know he is the "injured one," but I am injured, too.
> I have just lost my best friend.
> I don't even recognize the person who sleeps next to me now.
> —*Woman whose spouse has severe brain damage*

Compassion Fatigue is defined as a state of exhaustion and disfunction *[sic]*—biologically, psychologically, and socially—as a result of prolonged exposure to Compassion Stress and all that it evokes. It is a form of burnout. In families, this can lead to family conflict, disruption, and even divorce.

> —*Charles R. Figley*

> This is way over our heads.
> —*Family member*

> Chronic illness and disability are like thieves.
> They steal from two victims:
> the ill person and his or her caregiver.
> —*Lilly Cohen*

Alzheimer's disease (AD) is a progressive, fatal illness that afflicts more than four million Americans, ravaging its victims' minds for up to ten or more years…because of the long term burdens on them and the potential physical and emotional consequences, family members are recognized as the secondary victims of AD.

> —*Carol Williams and Brenda Moretta*

> Traumatized families are those who are attempting
> to cope with an extraordinary stressor
> that has disrupted their normal life routine.
>
> *—Charles R. Figley*

Secondary traumatic stress (STS) is the experience of tension and distress directly related to the demands of living with and caring for someone who displays the symptoms of post-traumatic stress disorder (PTSD).

—Charles R. Figley

Family burnout is defined here as the ultimate fatigue of intimate relationships…a family that has suffered fatigue associated with devotion to various family relationships that failed to produce the expected rewards.

—Charles R. Figley

> Burnout…state of physical, emotional,
> and mental exhaustion caused by long-term involvement
> in emotionally demanding situations.
>
> *—A. Pines and E. Aronson*

> I just don't have anything left!
>
> *—Parent of a child with ADHD*

Compassion Stress is defined as
the stress connected with exposure to a sufferer.

—*Charles R. Figley*

Somebody, HELP!

—*Family member*

I'm not crazy after all! For a while, I thought it was all me—
something I was doing wrong.
Now I know it is much bigger than that. What a relief!

—*Family member*

To understand everything is to forgive everything.

—*French proverb*

A truth that's told with a bad intent
bests all the lies you can invent.

—*Sufi expression*

Acknowledging the reality of trauma and traumatic reactions changes
the lives of all family members.

—*Charles R. Figley*

The inevitable stresses of family life in general, combined with the particular patterns of past and current adaptation, are now examined in attempts to understand how environments may exacerbate or mitigate preexisting biological or genetic vulnerabilities or current stresses. In this process, an increased respect is developing for the reciprocal of processes of influence between patients and their families. In addition to the long-recognized impact of families on individuals, there is an increased recognition of the impact of dysfunctional patients on their families—including the impact of the cumulative stress and burden of coping with chronic problems.

—Froma Walsh and Carol Anderson

It matters less what type of disease the patient has
than what type of patient has the disease.

—Hippocrates

Nothing clutters the soul more than remorse, resentment, recrimination. Negative feelings occupy a fearsome amount of space in the mind, block our perceptions, our prospects, our pleasures.

—Norman Cousins

There is no object so foul that intense light will not make it beautiful.

—Ralph Waldo Emerson

To be surprised, to wonder, is to begin to understand.

—José Ortega y Gasset

Chapter 3: The Diagnoses

> Just when the caterpillar thought the world was over,
> it became a beautiful butterfly.
>
> —*Saying on greeting card*

Now that we have a better realization, and perhaps acceptance, that life is difficult and that our problems require identification, or diagnosis, in order to heal, we can better appreciate the plight of all members of the family. It is important to note, though, that we are still very much in the beginning stages of truly understanding a great many of our problems. In the meantime, we will have to be patient with our ability to make diagnoses, realizing their limitations as well as their advantages. When done mindfully, with discipline and presence, they can offer much.

Before a diagnosis is made—and it is not that uncommon for the correct diagnosis to take years to emerge—the individual and the family are more likely to feel victimized rather than heroic; they are more likely to act unconsciously and mindlessly rather than consciously and mindfully; they are more likely to be shame-based rather than self-esteem based; they are more likely to personalize much of life as if life is all about them rather than seeing the universal in the most particular situation; and they are more prone to addictions and compulsions.

In addition, family members are likely to find that their immune system is compromised, their physical health stretched, and their emotional well being threatened. Probably, they are exposed to more dangerous accidents, too. In addition, they all are more likely to have a host of other wounds. Wounds never travel alone. There is an old expression, "Injury begets injury," meaning that once injured, you have an increased probability of being injured again. It is as if you become a magnet, attracting all kinds of other problems. None of this is your fault; all of this is your responsibility. Until you are accountable to your illness, or the impact of someone else's illness, you are its slave. Invisible problems remain invincible.

Healing begins with a diagnosis and ends when the diagnosis is no longer an issue or even important. First things first, though. In order to deal with wounds more effectively, it is time to look closer at the underbelly of these problems. It is time to examine more thoroughly the nature of the injury to all members of the family.

As we access our wounds, many questions arise. What is the nature of a wound? Where do they come from? What behaviors, attitudes, or symptoms do they cause? Is there any positive value to them? How can we respond or treat them? Are there guides to help us? How do we get started and move forward? Like problems, is there a wound or are there wounds? The following chapter addresses these vital concerns.

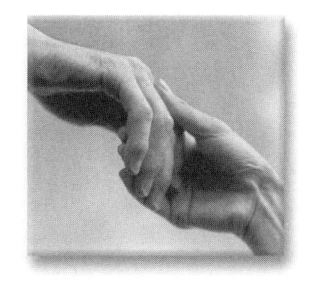

CHAPTER 4

The Wound

There are many different kinds of wounds that we can incur. They may be overt or obvious to virtually everyone who witnesses them. There are also covert wounds, the insults and injuries that are not so readily seen. I have witnessed both types of wounds—the often devastating effects of the problems and diagnoses described in the last two chapters on the mind, body, and spirit of those people that I have seen in the laboratory of my consultation office, workshops, and seminars.

Wherever there are problems that result in diagnoses, there are people with wounds. Wounds are important to recognize because they make real our problems that underlie diagnoses. More to the point, understanding the nature of the wound opens the doors to healing.

The type of wound is often important, particularly its "acceptability," or the degree of entitlement the person has to his or her pain, whether bestowed by society or granted by the person himself or herself. Ours is a culture that generally has little tolerance for wounding of most kinds, especially emotional wounds. Surveys show that there is still much stigma to being ill, especially illness that involves the mind. What is more, ours is a society that values emotional toughness over vulnerability, and individualism over collectivism.

Wounds that are of human design are often especially severe and long lasting. The impact of the wound is a complex interaction among three variables: the kind and severity of the incident or trauma, the resources of the person, and the response the person receives from his or her environment.

There are physical wounds, which are wounds to the body; psychological wounds, which include emotional and mental injuries; and spiritual wounds, which injure our ability to connect with a force or presence that is beyond everyday life. It is common for a person to have more than one type of wound. For example, a person can be sexually abused, which means the person most likely experienced physical trauma from the assault; emotional trauma from the feelings of guilt, betrayal, inferiority, and poor self-esteem, to name but a few; and spiritual abuse because of the power differential that typically exists when this type of wound occurs.

Physical wounding is the easiest to recognize. These wounds breach the physical integrity of the body. They break through the outermost layer of the body as they penetrate the skin. Psychological or spiritual wounds, while less visible, penetrate the emotional body. They can be defined as any injury to the self. The self is that part of us that organizes, sequences, and makes sense out of our experiences. Without a sense of self, we have little idea who we are, or what we stand for. Like leaves blown helter skelter in the wind, we become like leaves blown in life's storm. With a sense of self, on the other hand, the opportunity for life to become meaningful, full and enjoyable ensues.

The deepest wounds cause a type of bankruptcy, a loss of self, and ultimately a kind of soul murder. Major wounds assault and disrupt our assumptions about life. Our assumptions give our life meaning, stability, and security. When we are severely wounded, we no longer feel invincible, but rather feel powerless in a meaningless and insignificant world; in addition, we may feel that bad or evil forces surround us. What is more, we may feel bad about ourselves, thinking that there is something wrong with us, as if the wound were somehow our fault. We begin to feel shame and guilt for what has happened to us, and we can come to believe the worst about ourselves. As noted, society can be of little help.

Wounds that are deep change us forever. It's as if we turn a corner, and when we look back, we don't ever see the world, or our life, as we once did. Something forever changes when we receive a major wound. Remember the fish pond metaphor? Before a wound, it is as if we have been swimming in a fish pond that is familiar. We know where the rocks are and where and what the other fish are. We know the temperature of the water, the feel of the water, even the taste of the water. There are not too many surprises in our safe pond.

The deeper the wound, the less whole is the self. More fragmentation is present in the person. With fragmentation, the person is out of control. He or she can think one thing, feel another, and do a third. The result is a type of chaos that defeats healing and triumph.

> Tragedy: a serious drama typically describing
> a conflict between the protagonist and a superior force
> and having a sorrowful or disastrous conclusion.
>
> —Webster's New Collegiate Dictionary

> A catastrophe is an extraordinary event or series of events
> which is sudden, overwhelming, and often dangerous,
> either to one's self or significant other(s).
>
> —Charles R. Figley

God, this hurts. What happened to my baby?
—*Family member of a child with a neurobiological disorder*

Obstacles are those frightful things you see
when you take your eyes off your goal.
—*Henry Ford*

Hell is the suffering of being unable to love.
—*Dostoevsky*

A sinner is a soul enclosed in the prison of the self.
—*William J. Everett*

Illness, like death, is a universal experience;
there is no privilege that can make us immune to its touch.
—*Kat Duff*

The Boggle threshold—the level in your mind
where new ideas are so threatening that you snap.
—*Family member*

There is no right way to do a wrong thing.
—*Norman Vincent Peale*

The rules in the alcoholic's family:

1. The dependent's use of alcohol is the most important thing in the family's life.
2. Alcohol is not the cause of the family's problem.
3. Someone or something else caused the alcoholic's dependency; he is not responsible.
4. The status quo must be maintained at all cost.
5. Everyone in the family must be an 'enabler.'
6. No one may discuss what is really going on in the family, either with one another or with outsiders.
7. No one may say what he is feeling.

—*Sharon Wegscheider*

With the fearful strain on me night and day,
if I did not laugh I should die.

—*Abraham Lincoln*

What victims most commonly seek is vindication. They want public acknowledgment that what happened to them was wrong. They want the burden of shame lifted from their shoulders and placed where it belongs.

—*Judith Herman*

A victim explains his or her inability to cope
based on being victimized by a catastrophe,
while a survivor explains why he or she is able to cope
so effectively based on surviving a catastrophe.

—*Charles R. Figley*

What did I do to deserve this?
—*Family member*

The greatest abuse is to be treated as an object, to be put out of one's heart. It is this preexisting condition that allows all cruelty and abuse to occur. Without seeing someone as an object, as "another," intentional abuse cannot occur.
—*Stephen Levine*

Death is not the greatest loss in life;
the greatest loss is what dies inside us while we live.
—*Norman Cousins*

The longer we dwell on our misfortunes,
the greater is their power to harm us.
—*Voltaire*

Illness is telling us what we need to stop doing. If we look at illness that way, then it has great value. It might be telling us that we need to modify our work habits, to rest, or to question what we are doing.... It forces us to reach out for help, bring more love to us.
—*O. Carl Simonton*

What you are afraid of overtakes you.
—*Estonian proverb*

Chapter 4: The Wound

> The essence of psychological trauma is the loss of faith that there is order and continuity in life. Trauma occurs when one loses the sense of having a safe place to retreat within or outside oneself to deal with frightening emotions or experiences.
>
> —*Bessel A. van der Kolk*

> Man takes a drink, drink takes a drink,
> and drink takes the man.
>
> —*Japanese proverb*

> Denial is like a wall of fog that blinds us from seeing the truth. If you are a caregiver to someone with cancer, you are a hero—but if the person has a mental illness, you are suspect.
>
> —*Family member*

> Love is the burning point of life, and since all life is sorrowful, so is love. The stronger the love, the more the pain.
>
> —*Margaret Bourke-White*

> A man who fears suffering
> is already suffering from what he fears.
>
> —*Montage*

> Should we tell Johnny's teacher that he has a mental illness?
>
> —*Family member*

Mommy, aren't I important, too?
—*Daughter and sibling of someone with a neurobiological disorder*

There comes a time...when the "if only's" ring false
and the "why me's?" are boring.
To persist after that point is psychic death.
—Marion Woodman

...post-traumatic stress following victimization is largely due to the shattering of [three] basic assumptions victims hold about themselves and their world [i.e., the belief in personal invulnerability, the perception of the world as meaningful, and the perception of oneself as positive].... Coping...is presented as a process that involves rebuilding one's assumptive world.
—Ronnie Janoff-Bulman

Both of my parents abandoned me,
and they never left the house.
—*Adult child of two alcoholic parents*

Trauma itself doesn't produce pathology—
much of the insanity and despair you experience
comes directly from trying to manage
and control what you cannot.
—Herb Gravitz

It is likely that certain childhood experiences make people vulnerable to disorders of these neurotransmitter systems, which may later be activated under stress, particularly after the loss of affiliative bonds.

—*Bessel A. van der Kolk*

Caregiving is a high-stress activity.

—*Family member*

It is the social support between family members that prevents PTSD and secondary-traumatic stress disorder symptoms and any ongoing disruptions in the family structure and organization.

—*Herb Gravitz*

Disruption or loss of social support
is intimately associated with inability
to overcome the effects of psychological trauma.

—*Bessel A. van der Kolk*

Psychic trauma occurs when an individual is exposed to an overwhelming event resulting in helplessness in the face of intolerable danger, anxiety, and instinctual arousal.

—*Robert S. Pynoos and Spencer Eth*

Shit happens!

—*From the movie* Forrest Gump

The stressed person is less deleteriously affected if he or she:
1) perceives the event correctly; 2) translates the perceptions into a clear meaning; 3) relates the meaning to one's enduring attitude; 4) decides on appropriate action; and 5) revises memories, attitudes, and belief systems to fit new developmental lines made necessary by the experience.

—Mardi Jon Horowitz

A major difference between care and cure is that cure implies the end of trouble…but care has a sense of ongoing attention. There is no end. Conflicts may never be fully resolved.

—Thomas Moore

Until recently, the consequence of specific traumas…were generally considered separate entities. However, closer examination makes it clear that the human response to overwhelming and uncontrollable life events [trauma] is remarkably consistent.

—Bessel A. van der Kolk

I must go down!
I must go down deeper than ever I descended—
deeper into pain than ever I descend….
Thus my destiny wants it.

—Friedrich Nietzsche

If you can't feel pain, you can't feel anything.

—From the movie Ordinary People

Six factors apparently affect the long-term adjustment to traumatization: 1) the severity of the stressor, 2) genetic predisposition, 3) developmental phase, 4) a person's social support system, 5) prior traumatization, 6) preexisting personality.

—Bessel A. van der Kolk

The trauma syndrome is actually a continuous range of reaction. In addition to the classic biphasic alternation of denial and intrusion …there are two other long-term effects: secondary elaboration and post-traumatic decline. Secondary elaboration is a characterological adaptation to traumatization that includes depression, avoidance of intimacy, and "relational distortions." Post-traumatic decline is an impoverishment of activity and role functioning secondary to psychological constriction and phobic avoidance.

—Steven Krugman

Nature is waves: crest and trough, summer and winter, ebb and flow. Nature is circles: day and night, evaporation and rain, turn and return. Nature is made up of seemingly opposed but actually complementary energies that alternate and wax and wane like the moon.

—Robert and Jane Alter

Clinically, however, the most common pathological outcome of traumatic experiences are…dysthymia or major depression, dissociative reactions, anxiety disorders, adjustment reactions, substance abuse as self-medication, and personality alteration.

—John P. Wilson

Suicide is a final answer to a temporary problem.
—*Family member*

It is well established in the research and treatment literature that families can be the context for victimization.... Families traumatized from intrafamily abuse are often the most difficult to detect and treat.
—*Charles R. Figley*

Life is a lot like a motion picture.
When trauma happens, though, life becomes like a snapshot. The movement stops and everything freezes.
—*Family member*

All people suffer loss. Being alive means suffering loss. Sometimes the loss is natural, predictable, and even reversible.... But there is a different kind of loss that inevitably occurs in all of our lives.... This kind of loss has more devastating results, and it is irreversible. Such loss includes terminal illness, disability, divorce, rape, emotional abuse, physical and sexual abuse, chronic unemployment, crushing disappointment, mental illness, and ultimately death. If normal, natural, reversible loss is like a broken limb, then catastrophic loss is like an amputation. The results are permanent, the impact incalculable, the consequences cumulative.
—*Gerald L. Sittser*

What is to give light must endure burning.
—*Viktor Frankl*

Chapter 4: The Wound

> All the world is full of suffering;
> it is also full of overcoming it.
>
> —Helen Keller

Mourning is a process of sharing the many feelings one has over a loss. The family needs to create an atmosphere in which mourning is encouraged.

—Herb Gravitz

Although chronic and life-threatening illnesses of any sort will generate confusion, ambiguity, complexity, and anxiety about setting proper boundaries with a sick person, these problems are compounded in the case of mental illness. For example, rarely will patients question the diagnosis of such serious physical illnesses as cancer or heart disease. In contrast, those diagnosed with depression, manic-depression, or schizophrenia often vigorously deny the disease label. Unlike most physical illnesses, caregivers to the mentally ill (especially parents) must often contend with the possibility that they are somehow implicated in the creation of the other's problem. Finally, despite their best efforts, caregivers are sometimes treated as though they were an enemy by their loved one.

—David A. Karp

> When the heart weeps for what it has lost
> The Soul rejoices for what it has found.
>
> —Sufi expression

Worse still is the death of the spirit, the death that comes through guilt, regret, bitterness, hatred, immorality, and despair. The first kind of death happens to us; the second kind of death happens in us. It is a death we bring upon ourselves if we refuse to be transformed by the first death.

—*Gerald L. Sittser*

Great loss of whatever kind is always bad,
only bad in different ways.

—*Family member*

Our consciousness can evolve only if we are willing
to risk looking for the meaning of our lives
as rigorously as we adapt to the world in which we live.

—*Paul Pearsall*

Our culture promotes very negative attitudes toward illness, as if being unwell were some sign of weakness or a personal shortcoming. People are made to feel ashamed of being sick, especially if they are seriously ill, and this can lead one to feel guilty about being ill even to despise oneself for being ill.

—*Morrie Schwartz*

He that lacks time to mourn, lacks time to mend.

—*William Shakespeare*

> No problem can be solved from the same consciousness
> that created it. We must learn to see the world anew.
> —*Albert Einstein*

> Suffering is always some form of nonacceptance,
> some form of unconscious resistance to what is.
> —*Herb Gravitz*

> I feel ashamed for being ill—for being human.
> —*Person with ALS*

Entropy is a concept that predicts that everything and everyone is in the process of falling apart and burning up. As violent as this sounds, entropy is, in fact, a process and not a verdict regarding our existence. Entropy is really a positive and necessary for that is one aspect of our movement through the chaos of living. We are only falling apart so we fall together again in a different and higher order.

—*Paul Pearsall*

> Compulsions give you a false sense of pleasure,
> pleasure that always turns to pain.
> —*Recovering alcoholic*

> I never ever, in my wildest dreams,
> thought that I would wind up here.
> —*Man waiting for a kidney transplant*

> Reality is when it happens to you.
> —*Bumper sticker*

> If there is a sin against life,
> it consists perhaps not so much in despairing of life
> as in hoping for another life
> and eluding the implacable grandeur of this life.
> —*Albert Camus*

Despite a backdrop of denial and minimization, the doors to healing and triumphing over the wounds of all the participants in the family experience are opening. Just as we have painfully and reluctantly recognized the pain of alcoholism on the family as well as the alcoholic, we are now recognizing the effects of our other wounds on the entire family.

Wounding is an interpersonal process as well as an intrapsychic, or inside the person, experience. It does not occur in isolation from the larger aspects of life. Wounds occur and unfold in the context of social situations. And the most important social situation is the family. Only now is the full impact of this beginning to be realized.

The family is the major shock absorber between the individual and the rest of the world. It may be the only place where any of us are not replaceable. When one member incurs a problem, all members can suffer. Consequently, when any member of the family is affected, everyone is affected. There is little escape from wound's wake—only the desire, the effort, and the determination not only to prevail, but also actually to triumph—not despite the wound but because of it.

Wounds injure the core of the self, that part of us that gives order and meaning to our lives. Interestingly, though, the type and nature of the wound are often not the primary determinants of healing. More and more attention is being given to the resources of the person and the resources in the person's environment as determinants of the wound's impact. It is to this topic of the broader impact of our wounds that we now turn, for the deeper the wound, the deeper the impact.

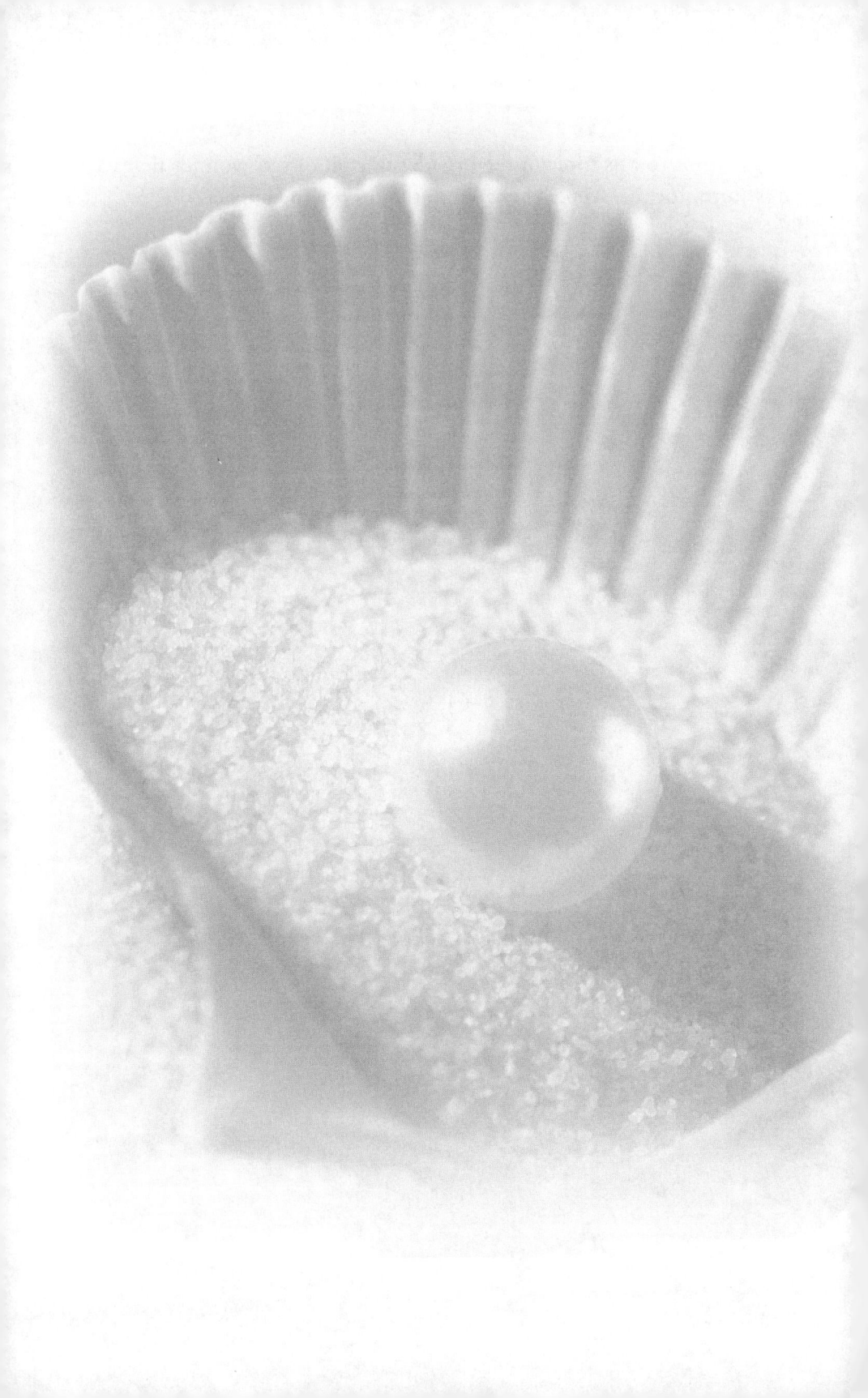

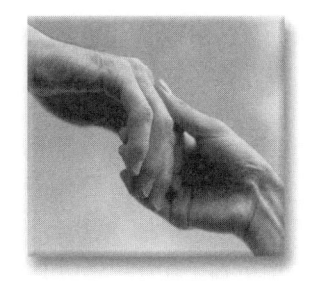

CHAPTER 5

The Impact of the Wound

Wounds have direct and indirect effects. Most obvious is the wound to the direct sufferer. As we have seen, the direct sufferer is the one on whom the wound is perpetrated or inflicted. He or she is the direct symptom bearer. Understandably, this member of the family has received the most attention.

The primary sufferer incurs a wound that is typically recognizable and often visible. Their wounds are apparent; they are obvious. There is blood that has been shed—literally or figuratively. Few would deny the existence of the wound, although sadly many try to obliterate its presence through denial, which is a very primitive refusal to recognize the reality of a situation. Nevertheless, these direct sufferers are typically shamed, stigmatized, and marginalized by a society that often has little tolerance for the wounded.

But what is less known and even less accepted is that there is almost always an invisible sufferer for every visible sufferer. In fact, it has been suggested that there are between four and six people affected by every one sufferer. These "hidden" sufferers are the secondary sufferers. They are the family, the loved ones, and the friends of the primary sufferer. I refer to them as "the neglected affected" in my other writings.

The bottom line is that a problem between two people never belongs to just one of them.

Often the plight of the secondary sufferers is no less painful. Typically, they suffer in silence. Families can be six times punished: they are often forced to watch the deterioration of a loved one, they are blamed for the problem instead of trained, they are isolated from others—often shunned—they are often excluded from treatment, and, adding insult to injury, they are often forced to pay for their loved one's treatment. They, too, are often stigmatized. Given our society's predilection to ignore and deny problems in the first place, it should be of little surprise that the impact of their problems is denied and ignored even more!

In the book *Mental Illness and the Family: Unlocking the Doors to Triumph,* I describe the five major ways that the secondary sufferers are affected. They experience impending stress and frequent trauma, unrelenting sadness and ever-present loss, chronic sorrow and ongoing grief, widespread guilt, and constant fatigue and persistent exhaustion. These five characteristics typically apply to all of those who are under the influence of any serious, severe, and chronic illness, addiction, or other trauma. In addition, each member of the family can experience wounding differently. Thus, the parents, the children, the spouse, the siblings, and members of the extended family can each have their own special wounds because each has his or her own unique role or function in the family. It goes without saying that in addition to the universal signs of family distress, each separate diagnosis presents its own distinctive challenges.

Secondary sufferers must break away from the emotional roller coaster of pain, powerlessness, shame, guilt, confusion, fear, disappointment, exhaustion, and frustration that is so often their lot. Leaving loved ones to their own fate may be one of the most difficult of all undertakings for the secondary sufferer. While this statement, of course, is dependent upon the age of the sufferer and his or her current soundness, it is nonetheless important. Even children have their own destiny.

Healing involves recognition, validation, and help to both populations of sufferers. To that end, the plight of all members of the family must be addressed. In the next series of sayings, we will look at the common denominators among primary sufferers and secondary sufferers as well as distinguish the two from each other. While both can show similar effects, the approach to healing and recovery can be very different. Their needs can be different. And so can their treatment.

> Then I realized exactly the situation—
> my life did depend on it.
> —*Erin Brockovich*

It's morning in Manhattan. A woman pushes a man in a wheelchair to a curb. She hails a cab. She opens the cab door. He stands shakily and she helps him in. She folds up the chair. She stashes it in front. She walks around the cab and gets in beside him. Do you think? A.) Oh, the poor man, or B.) Oh, the poor woman.

—*Maggie Strong*

> Our house was like a constant fire drill.
> —*Family member*

> There is a cost to caring.
> —*Charles R. Figley*

Seeing someone you love suffer from a major mental illness [or any serious illness] is an extremely painful, frightening, confusing, and infuriating experience.

—*Rebecca Woolis*

My grief is like a funeral that never ends
and nobody cares about.

—*Family member*

Disenfranchised grief is grief that cannot be
openly acknowledged, socially shared,
or publicly supported.

—*Kenneth Doka*

Recovery must include the family, too.

—*Herb Gravitz*

I feel like I have been cheated out of
a lot of the good things in life.

—*Family member*

Even Gandhi would yell and scream if he had my child.

—*Family member*

On any given evening I might hear about the unimaginable pain surrounding the decision to have a child removed from one's home by the police, the powerlessness of visiting a spouse or child in a hospital who is so muddled by powerful medication that he or she can barely speak, the shame that accompanies hating someone you love because of what their illness has done to you and your family, the guilt that lingers from the belief that you might somehow be responsible for another person's descent into mental illness, the confusion associated with navigating the Byzantine complexities of the mental health system, the fear associated with waiting for the next phone call announcing yet another suicide attempt by someone close to you, the disappointment that a talented son or daughter may never realize even a fraction of their potential, the exhaustion that accompanies full-time caregiving, or the frustration of being unable to take even a brief vacation. Pain, powerlessness, shame, guilt, confusion, fear, disappointment, exhaustion, frustration: these emotions are the currency of conversation among the Family and Friends group members.

—David A. Karp

Everything about family life changes
when a family member becomes mentally ill.

—E. Farrell and J. Murphy

You expect me to be private about carrying the burden of your illness. I know it is embarrassing and shameful to you, but I have to share this and get my own help.

—Family member

Every illness, minor or major,
is a crucible that tries our metal and tests our limits.

—*Kat Duff*

When your spouse or partner is diagnosed
with a serious chronic illness or disability,
you become a caregiver.

—*Well Spouse Foundation*

I had to leave!
I left the relationship because I thought I was losing my mind
and my own health was at risk.
I wasn't helping or making a difference anyway.

—*Spouse*

The illness can become the central organizing principle
around which the family operates.

—*Herb Gravitz*

There can be no greater trauma than helplessly watching your loved one permanently, irretrievably, and, in most cases, unwillingly being pulled away; knowing the terror that the unknown can bring; forcing oneself to come to closure with that loved one; seeing the robbing of that loved one's personal control and the massive violations of his or her assumptive world.

—*Therese A. Rando*

So you want to know what it takes to live with this illness?
It's like having the problems of Job,
which require the wisdom of Solomon,
the strength of Hercules, the patience of Mother Teresa,
the Midas touch, and Gandhi's temperament.

—*Family member*

The behaviors associated with severe mental illnesses, such as delusions, hallucinations, manic fervor, impaired judgement, poor handling of money, lapses in grooming, obsessions, even apathy and withdrawal, can be highly disturbing and often embarrassing to you and your family members.

—*Rosalynn Carter*

One moment my child's illness is like a bully, picking on him.
The next, it is a bully picking on us.

—*Family member*

Like the four characters in Rashomon, parents, children, siblings, and spouses have different perceptions and experiences of everything affecting the life of a family. In large part, these differences arise from the distinctive roles each performs in the family's emotional, economic, and practical division of labor.

—*David A. Karp*

The illness is like an octopus.
It has its tentacles around every one of us!

—*Family member*

Each long-term illness has its own dynamics, and each individual or family system is likely to live out its challenges in particular ways. But for children and adolescents, there are often issues such as those related to responsibility (Did I cause Grandpa's cancer?), blame (Did Uncle Ted's AIDS result from his life style?), and guilt (Did I wish my father would get it over with and die so that the rest of us could go back to our normal life?).

—*Charles A. Corr*

The field of traumatology has inadvertently ignored a large segment of traumatized people: the family and other supporters of "victims." In other words, we have ignored those suffering in their own right as a result of a loved one being traumatized.

—*Charles R. Figley*

It was like someone kidnapped our boy.
The person we grew to know and love was gone!

—*Family member*

Caregivers are the other halves of illness experiences.

—*Arthur Frank*

This is just one big sinkhole and it is depleting everyone.
I know I shouldn't be, but I am plain angry.

—*Family member*

Learned helplessness is the giving-up reaction, the quitting response that follows from the belief that whatever you do doesn't matter.... [It is] caused by experience in which subjects learned that nothing they did mattered and that their responses didn't work to bring them what they wanted. This experience taught them to expect that, in the future, and in new situations, their actions would once again be futile. Learned helplessness seemed to be at the core of defeat and failure. We knew the cause of learned helplessness, and now we could see it as the cause of depression: the belief that your actions will be futile.

—Martin P. Seligman

Serious mental illness is a catastrophic stressor
that can leave families traumatized and debilitated.

—Diane Marsh

Did I cause it? Is it my fault?
Will I catch it? Who will take care of me?

—*Young child and sibling of a person with a neurobiological disorder*

I just dread telling anyone about the illness. Almost everyone responds with their favorite theory about what I did—or didn't do—that brought it on. I don't know if it's worse, but most also have their theories about how to make things better.

—*Cancer survivor*

When one finger hurts, soon the whole hand hurts.
And then the whole arm.
And before you know it, the whole body hurts.

—*Philip Benjamin Gravitz*

There ought to be a support group
for us poor bastards (spouses), too.

—*Spouse*

Time and again, family members raise questions about closeness and distance, independence and dependence, giving one's self to others fully or preserving themselves by disengaging. Line drawing is part of every discussion about coping because of the inevitable feeling that wherever they have drawn the line it is the 'wrong' place. To give money or to withhold it? To allow a child to live at home or…independently? To accept a spouse's failure…or insist that they exercise greater personal responsibility? To rescue…or let them struggle…. These are the kinds of questions that cause caregiving agony.

—*David A. Karp*

Too many of the doctors didn't even mention sex.
And they are relieved when we didn't, too.
But we needed to talk to someone.

—*Married couple under the influence of antidepressants*

Do we tell John's teacher?

—*Parent of a child with a neurobiological disorder*

To become chronically ill is to lose yourself as a healthy person: you grieve. To be married to someone ill and to watch a man or woman you love suffer means you mourn. You mourn the lost marriage, the lost family, the suffering of the mate, and your lost self.

—*Maggie Strong*

What will everybody think? Will they blame us?

—*Parents of a child with a neurobiological disorder*

I not only had to downsize my expectations for my ill child, but I had to ratchet down my own life expectations. That is insult to injury!

—*Family member*

Not only is it better for the sick to be left alone at times, it is also better for the well to leave them at times. Healthy people can be contaminated by the gloom and depression of the ailing if they come too close or have too much sympathy.

—*Kat Duff*

At first they asked how we were all doing. Then they asked how our ill son was doing. They still ask about him—but less. But now they never ask about us. We're starting to feel that we don't exist anymore.

—*Parents of a mentally ill child*

When you finally get to be a grown up,
you know how small and powerless you really are.

—*Spouse*

It's a double whammy. First you become a superwoman or a superman. Then you become invisible. The ill person becomes number one and you become number two. Soon you don't become anyone.

—*Family member*

How do we tell our other children that their brother is mentally ill? How do we tell our friends? Should we tell our relatives? Who do we tell—and when? It's all so confusing.

—*Parents of a mentally ill child*

I have no feelings left.
My face had become a no-see and no-feel mask.
I am devastated.

—*Spouse of a man fighting cancer*

First, I felt confused when our daughter was diagnosed with an NBD. Then, I felt angry at her. Then, I felt guilty. Finally, I felt so ashamed for having all of those feelings.

—*Parent of a child with a neurobiological disorder*

The family is overloaded and undersupported.

—*Herb Gravitz*

> What about our pain, too!
> No one knows how hard it has been
> these last ten years since our son became ill.
>
> —*Parents of a man with a neurobiological disorder*

Some illnesses come and go in bouts: ulcerative colitis and certain cancers and perhaps two-thirds of the cases of multiple sclerosis. Unpredictable stable periods alternate with unpredictable flare-ups. The family must master two gears: the "well" gear when they act relatively normal and the "sick" gear when options close tight around the illness.

> —*Maggie Strong*

> I don't think I've felt rested any time in the last fifteen years!
>
> —*Parent of a child with severe allergies who suffers anaphylaxis*

> You just can't imagine the burdens,
> the shame and the complexity of this unless you live it.
>
> —*Family member*

Doctors and nurses often instruct us in how to make the patient's life easier. Psychotherapists detail the patient's fear. Physiotherapists explain how to move a patient's ankle or an elbow painlessly. But for us? Nada. We don't have a name. We don't even know our own needs.

> —*Maggie Strong*

> It's like I am in the middle of a big storm.
> Just about when you think it's about to die down,
> something else pops up.
>
> —*Family member*

The primary dialectic (tension) between the family and the sufferer is between caring and freedom—the line between my need to take care of you and my need to take care of me. This is the fundamental dilemma and the fundamental ambivalence and this arises from two powerful and contradictory cultural messages: one is to love, protect, and care for family members regardless of the personal cost and the second is that we have the right—indeed the responsibility—to pursue personal happiness and fulfilment.

—*David A. Karp*

By definition, the effects of vicarious traumatization on an individual resemble those of traumatic experiences. They included significant disruption in one's sense of meaning, connection, identity, and world view, as well as in one's affect [emotion] tolerance, psychological needs, beliefs about self and others, interpersonal relationships, and sensory memory, including imagery.

—*Charles R. Figley*

> I can't believe that I married another alcoholic.
> He only drank a case of beer each weekend.
>
> —*Spouse and daughter of an alcoholic*

The most important variable, that may "encode" a trauma—which may determine whether there will actually be traumatization—may well be the person's perception of the traumatic event. Perception of the event in many cases is more important than actual circumstance. Put differently, the subjective appraisal of the event is often more important than the objective nature of the event itself.

—*Herb Gravitz*

We've lost our sense of normalcy.

—*The family of a child with schizophrenia*

When you have got an elephant by the hind legs and he is trying to run away, it's best to let him run.

—*Abraham Lincoln*

The extent of children's anxieties in reaction to the bombing in London during World War II was associated with their parents' reaction rather than with their exposure to the bombing itself. [It is] similarly observed [that] children's reactions to bombardment on kibbutzim in Israel [are] determined more by their parents' attitudes than by the intensity of the danger experienced.

—*Charles R. Figley*

Suicide is when someone hangs his or her skeleton in your closet.

—*Adult survivor of a family member's suicide*

The family perception of crisis is a major influencing factor in how a family will respond to crisis. Ultimately, it is proposed that in chronic illness, the crisis is not the problem, but it is the family's constraining beliefs that restrict alternative views about the crisis that become the problem.

—*Drs. Shaw and Halliday*

First I lost my wife to her illness. I lost my partner. Then I lost our sexual relationship. Then I lost many of our friends, who couldn't take it anymore. Then I lost most of our savings and retirement. Then I lost our future. I have to make all the big decisions alone. And now I have lost our marital equality.

—*Spouse of a person with a neurobiological disorder*

If we broaden our perspective beyond a dyadic bond and early life determinants, we become aware that resilience is woven in a web of relationships and experiences over the course of the life cycle and across the generations.

—*Froma Walsh*

No cultural factor has greater weight or sheer force in determining caregiving roles than gender. In general, when both genders are involved in caregiving, the following occurs:
1. Women take on greater responsibility than men do.
2. Mothers take on more responsibility than fathers do.
3. Wives take on greater responsibility than husbands do.
4. Sisters take on more responsibility than brothers do.

—*David A. Karp*

> I don't know who I am anymore.
>
> —*Family member*

Ill family members, or the primary sufferers, can always contribute in seven major ways:

1. Acknowledge that you have a problem.
2. Get treatment.
3. Stay in recovery.
4. Allow your loved ones to have their own feelings of hurt and injury, and take them no more personally than your behaviors toward them are personal. In other words, appreciate the impact.
5. Find ways to help out, regardless of how inconsequential they may seem.
6. Be accountable—to the illness, to yourself, to your family.
7. Remember, success is getting up one more time than you fall down—so hang in there and don't give up!

—*Herb Gravitz*

The emotional health of children in a family is affected by the emotional relationship between their parents. When the couple relationship is warm and supportive, children are more likely to be healthy and happy.

—*Herb Gravitz*

> I'll help you when I can, but only if you're helping yourself. Because if you're not going to do anything to help yourself, I can't help you either.
>
> —*Parent to his 25-year-old son*

Their findings [longitudinal studies of at-risk children] revealed that earlier researchers focused too narrowly on maternal influence and the damage of one parent in the nuclear household, and missed the importance of siblings and others [including pets, in my experience] in the extended family network.

—*Froma Walsh*

What good is quantifying loss? What good is comparing? The right question to ask is not, "Whose is worse?" It is to ask, "What meaning can be gained from suffering, and how can we grow through suffering?

—*Gerald L. Sittser*

Survivor guilt is a very common form of guilt among family members and trauma survivors. It is the feeling that we do not deserve to have a better life than those we love or even have a life.

—*Herb Gravitz*

I stopped trying to be heard because it made mom feel so bad.

—*Child of a mentally ill mother*

. . . the experience of loss itself does not have to be the defining moment of our lives. Instead, the defining moment can be our response to the loss. It is not what happens to us that matters as much as what happens in us.

—*Gerald L. Sittser*

At no point in my life did it occur to me that my many accidents (including fights, failed relationships, medical problems, and depression) were a consequence of my drinking. It was only after my alcoholism had been identified and treated that I was able to clearly see the path of carnage that alcoholism had cut though my life.

—Joseph Beasley

Man needs difficulties; they are necessary for health.

—Carl Jung

I had come to see falling apart, at least as far as depression was concerned, not so much as an unfortunate event, but often as a necessary prelude to personal renewal following significantly stressful events.

—Frederic Flach

Wounds are unavoidable. As one family member said, "We have no voting rights when it comes to being wounded, but we do have some choices." He went on to add: "The more healing, the more choices." Interestingly, I believe this is true—up to a point. I have found that as we, and as the family, move further and further into healing, the fewer choices there actually may be. This is because the choices become more and more clear as the consequences of these choices become more and more obvious. If, for example, my purpose is to have a clean diet, there are fewer choices to follow than if my intention is simply to eat.

We can lie back and utter, either loudly or quietly, that life is unfair, that this should have or should never have happened to us, and that we consequently have no choice but to suffer. We can take M. Scott Peck's "road less travelled," or Joseph Campbell's "hero or heroine's journey." We can transform our wound and make it "a sacred wound" as Jean Houston would point to, or we can create from our wounding what Baba Ram Dass calls "fierce grace." We might even find Nietzsche's "good enemy" in our traumas, addictions, and illnesses.

Regardless, the family, like any system, becomes altered in reaction to the traumatization of any member. In the resulting system, the world is no longer as benevolent, as kind, as just, or as controllable. Life often lacks purpose and meaning. Nothing is ever the same, and no one is as safe as he or she once was. As one family exclaimed: "Our world has been turned upside down." However, wounds come in many forms and the form will determine how both the primary and secondary sufferer will experience the wound.

Let us continue our trek by discerning the two basic forms of wounds. Our wounds can be "profane" or they can be "sacred." And what a difference the difference makes! The distinction becomes an entry point to our journey from shame to self-esteem, from victim to hero, from unconsciousness to consciousness, from personalizing to universalizing, and from addiction to spaciousness. It opens the door not only to healing but also to triumphing regardless of circumstance. For in addition to being unavoidable and inevitable, wounds are also potentially useful, even invaluable.

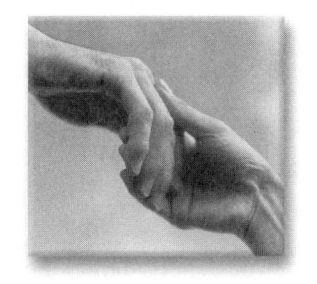

CHAPTER 6

Sacred and Profane Wounds

Wounds present themselves in two forms. Many of the wounds that we suffer are "profane wounds." These are wounds which make us ask: "Why me? What did I do to deserve this? What is wrong with me? Am I bad? Am I being punished?" We feel victimized by our life and our circumstances, in fact confounding the two, concluding that we are our situation instead of we have a situation, one that is so much smaller and limited than who we are. We confuse the part for the whole. We tend to personalize the injury, and feel like we are the only one who has such a hurt. We tend to isolate and withdraw from life. In the process, life becomes more meaningless, and we become emptier. Eventually, we lose contact not only with others, but also with our deeper selves and with our connection to a force or power beyond our physical, limited self.

Profane wounds invariably create shame as well as separation, and they are always an assault and affront to the ego, the small part of the psyche that loves to be in control and thinks it is the center of the universe. There is always struggle and little acceptance when the ego is involved. A profane wound is always full of drama. As one of my clients said, "We put our problems on a pedestal and worship 'em. That way, we don't have to do much."

A profane wound occurs when we "freeze frame" a particular—and usually horrible—scene. The event can involve someone we love or us. We are then stuck with that particular image or experience, and all of life becomes a constant replaying and reactivating of that one experience. That negative event is not only our past, but it becomes our future. It becomes the template upon which all new experience is projected.

On the other hand, when a wound becomes sacred, it is as if the frozen frames are able to move forward to now make a more complete story. As the movie evolves from frame to frame to frame, we get to see the whole of the movie, not just a small part. In the process we see, hear, and know things that were unavailable to us in that one, single episode. We struggle to find and make meaning for our negative experience now. We act responsibly and responsively. We waste little effort resisting, because we know that we need all of the energy we can bring to bear to the circumstance in order to have a life worth living and a loss worth enduring.

A sacred wound is a creative act. It is birthed by the soul instead of the ego. Rather than feeling like a victim who has no control over the circumstance, we accept the challenge of having mastery over how we respond. In the process, our struggle becomes elevated to the heroic. Instead of dwelling in our unconsciousness, we become more and more conscious. Instead of feeling alone and isolated, we feel connected to a larger universal pattern. Instead of shame, we feel self-esteem. Instead of addiction and crippling attachment, we feel spaciousness and freedom. And most important, a sacred wound enlarges our view of life, and lifts the small story of our explanation of what happened to a much larger and greater story, one in which we can find our place in the greater community or whole.

Having a sacred wound, we still feel the pain, and we still feel the injury. Nothing removes the pain. But sometimes, if we are open to the grace that is available to us all, we move forward in our pain, for how the pain is experienced is the crucial difference.

While both sacred and profane wounds injure us and while both may and do change us forever, one wound invites us to a deeper, more profound, and reverent view of life, while the other disempowers us. One opens the door to possibility; the other closes it. One allows us to embrace life; the other to avoid it.

> A Bird called the Phoenix
> One thousand years it lives,
> And at the end of those thousand years,
> Its nest is engulfed in flames, and consumes it.
> But the germ of its essence survives
> And renews itself and lives.
>
> —*Midrash Rabbah, Genesis, 19:5*

> People seldom tap into their deepest strengths and abilities until forced to do so by a major adversity.
>
> —*Al Siebert*

> Do you think that you shall enter the Garden of Bliss without such trials as come to those who passed before you?
>
> —*Koran*

> Life has meaning only in the struggle.
> Triumph or defeat is in the hands of the Gods....
> So let us celebrate the struggle!
>
> —*Swahili Warrior Song*

For the world is like an olive press, and men are constantly under pressure. If you are the dregs of the oil you are carried away through the sewer, but if you are true oil you remain in the vessel. To be under pressure is inescapable. Pressure takes place through all the world: war, siege, the worries of state. We all know men who grumble under these pressures, and complain. They are cowards. They lack splendor. But there is another sort of man who is under the same pressure, but does not complain. For it is the friction which polishes him. It is pressure which refines and makes him noble.

—*Saint Augustine*

I remind myself that tenacity is easier
when you have no choice.

—*Galen Rowell*

Perseverance is persisting, with grace, to glory.

—*American Oxford Dictionary, 2002*

There is no birth of consciousness without pain.

—*Carl Jung*

The shell must break before the bird can fly.

—*Alfred Lord Tennyson*

Chapter 6: Sacred and Profane Wounds

It is not good for all our wishes to be filled;
through sickness we recognize the value of health;
through evil, the value of good;
through hunger, the value of food;
through exertion, the value of rest.

—*Greek proverb*

Great truths come as complementary opposites.

—*Anonymous*

In every negative event
is the seed of an equal or greater benefit.

—*Napoleon Hill*

Religious man experiences two kinds of time—profane and sacred. The one is an evanescent duration, the other a "succession of eternities," periodically recoverable during the festivals that made up the sacred calendar. The liturgical time of the calendar flows in a closed circle; it is the cosmic time of the year, sanctified by the works of the gods.

—*Mircea Eliade*

Suffering is redemptive
when it leads us to a deeper,
more nuanced understanding
of ourselves and other humans.

—*Mary Pipher*

How strange would appear to be this thing that men call pleasure! And how curiously it is related to what is thought to be its opposite, pain!...Wherever the one is found, the other follows up behind.

—Plato

If God's justice could be recognized
as just by human comprehension,
it would not be divine.

—Martin Luther

Your limitations exist not to confine you, but to challenge you to greater and greater things. Those limitations give you a perfect platform against which to push ahead. Your limitations define your own special pathway to accomplishment. For in going beyond them you are moving forward in a truly meaningful way.

—Ralph Marston

By now you've figured out I'm into pain. Why? Because it's self-revelatory, that's why. There is a point in every race when a rider encounters his real opponent and understands that it's himself. In my most painful moments on the bike, I am at my most curious, and I wonder each and every time how I will respond. Will I discover my innermost weakness, or will I seek out my innermost strength? It's an open-ended question whether or not I will be able to finish the race. You might say pain is my chosen way of exploring the human heart.

— Lance Armstrong

> Make every obstacle an opportunity.
> Make every negative into a positive.
>
> —*Mother of Lance Armstrong*

> If this is a blessing, it is certainly well disguised.
>
> —*Winston Churchill*

> We rise to great heights by a winding staircase.
>
> —*Sir Francis Bacon*

> When you lose, don't lose the lesson.
>
> —*Dalai Lama*

> The ultimate measure of a man is not where he stands in moments of comfort and convenience, but where he stands at times of challenge and controversy.
>
> —*Martin Luther King, Jr.*

> What seems to be a great loss or punishment often turns out to be a lesson. I know, through my own experience, that God never closes one door without opening another.
>
> —*Yolande D. Herron*

> In the midst of a difficulty lies opportunity.
>
> —*Albert Einstein*

Self-confidence is the result
of a successfully survived risk.

—Jack Gibb

Nothing so concentrates experience
and clarifies the central conditions of living
as serious illness.

—Arthur Kleinman

The basic difference between an ordinary man and a warrior
is that a warrior takes everything as a challenge,
while an ordinary man takes everything
either as a blessing or a curse.

—Don Juan

Experience is not what happens to a man.
It is what a man does with what happens to him.

—Aldous Huxley

Objective life circumstances have a negligible role to play
in a theory of happiness.

—Richard Kammann

Life will either grind you down or polish you up,
and which it does is your choice.

—Roger Walsh

Stress is the test for goodness. The truly good are they who in time of stress do not desert their integrity, their maturity, their sensitivity. Nobility might be defined as the capacity not to regress in response to degradation, not to become blunted in the face of pain, to tolerate the agonizing and remain intact. As I have said elsewhere, "one measure and perhaps the best measure of a person's greatness is the capacity for suffering."

—*M. Scott Peck*

Myths, fairy tales, and great works of literature, which abound with cripples and hunchbacks, one-eyed monsters and big-nosed lovers, suggest that these abnormalities are not only normal, but somehow necessary in the plot of life; they shape our characters and destinies, forge our greatnesses and smallnesses, while entertaining and instructing others at the same time.

—*Kat Duff*

Eventually you may see the silver lining in the storm clouds [of mental illness]: increased awareness, sensitivity, receptivity, compassion, maturity, and [becoming] less judgmental, self-centered.

—*Rex Dickens*

The greatest treasure comes out of the most despised and secret places…. This place of greatest vulnerability is also a holy place, a place of healing….

—*Albert Kreinheder*

Somebody up there has decided to offer me another lesson.

—*Family member*

Tragedy brings forward the need to create meaning—
to tell new stories—that can reweave the frayed ends
of life into a coherent whole. Our ability to tell these stories
is positively linked with recovery....

—*Joan Borysenko*

Fearfulness is the first prerequisite of a spiritual life.

—*Mahatma Gandhi*

Lying deep in the depths of the human psyche is the sure knowledge that adversity is an essential component of any existence, if that existence is to be complete. The steel must be hardened, and the trial must be by fire if it is to be a trial at all. The mythic archetypes of all cultures represent this idea, enduring enormous physical onslaughts, pains, tortures, woundings—finally coming through, emerging greater and more complete than before—as the examples of Achilles, Prometheus, and Oedipus demonstrate in Western mythology.

—*Larry Dossey*

Age is opportunity no less
Than youth itself, though in another dress,
And as the evening twilight fades away
The sky is filled with stars invisible by day.

—*Henry Wadsworth Longfellow*

Chapter 6: Sacred and Profane Wounds

> Call the world, if you please,
> The veil of Soulmaking.
> Then you will find out
> The use of the world....
>
> —*John Keats*

Sacred psychology assumes that the deepest yearning in every human soul is to return to its spiritual source.... Through sacred psychology, you become a citizen in a universe larger than your aspiration and more complex than all your dreams.... Sacred psychology shows you that you are richer, deeper, stronger, and more a mystery than you know.... It elicits the evolutionary, latent codings within your body/mind/soul that have waited for tens of thousands of years to be activated....

—*Jean Houston*

> Sometimes I go about pitying myself,
> and all the time I am being carried on great winds across the sky.
>
> —*Chippewa saying*

> True illumination,
> like all real and vital experience,
> consists rather in the breathing of a certain atmosphere,
> the living at certain levels of consciousness,
> than in the acquirement of specific information.
>
> —*Evelyn Underhill*

In every adversity there are the seeds
of an equal or greater opportunity.

—*W. Clement Stone*

Great Story is like a force field, charging the many incidents of our personal history with meaning and significance. Great Story plays upon our minds like a symphony, activating different tones, themes, feelings, and fancies, illuminating parts of ourselves we didn't know we had.... Yet devastation, or at least radical surprise, is an inevitable and central theme of Great Story, which always engages us at our most fragile and wounded edges. Then, suddenly, in these events that wound, the ensuing holes make us holy.

—*Jean Houston*

The greatest guru of all is life.

—*Spouse of cancer survivor*

But never forget that you can only stumble if you're moving.

—*Richard Carlton*

Enlightenment is the end of suffering.

—*The Buddha*

Our daughter's illness is my worst nightmare and my greatest ecstasy.

—*Family member*

> I am so upset because he demands so much of my time
> and his treatment is so expensive.
>
> —*Spouse of a man with an NBD*

> Suffering has always been part of the maturation process
> of the saint and the mystic.
>
> —*Larry Dossey*

> Difficult experiences are very good training for the mind.
>
> —*Dalai Lama*

> Difficulties strengthen the mind, as labor does the body.
>
> —*Seneca*

> Confusion is a word we have invented
> for an order which is not yet understood.
>
> —*Henry Miller*

There is, thus, a collective statement from mystics of diverse sources that affirms the place in life for difficult, painful experience. Perfection of the spirit is, in fact, impossible to attain without it, we are told. Suffering, ill-health, and pain are not so much grotesque facts of life as they are prerequisites for the opening of the doors of perception. Without the conjoined fact of the good and the bad, of health and illness, there is no advance of the spirit, only stasis and stagnation.

—*Larry Dossey*

But suppose pleasure and pain were so linked together
that he who wants to have the greatest possible amount of the one
must have the greatest possible amount of the other also?

—*Friedrich Nietzsche*

Every difficulty in life presents us with an opportunity to turn inward and to invoke our own submerged inner resources. The trials we endure can and should introduce us to our strengths. Prudent people look beyond the incident itself and seek to form the habit of putting it to good use.

—*Epictetus*

Chaos is a time of great creativity and opportunity.
As the bricks of the past become unstuck and crumble,
there is the chance to rebuild in new and better ways.

—*F. Ogden*

In fact, I feel I am even more myself
than I was before I got this illness
because I have been able to transcend many of the psychological
and emotional limitations I had before I developed ALS.

—*Morrie Schwartz*

Do you think that you shall enter the Garden of Bliss
without such trials as come to those who passed before you?

—*Koran*

Chapter 6: Sacred and Profane Wounds

When one door of happiness closes, another opens;
but often we look so long at the closed door
that we do not see the one that has been opened for us.

—Helen Keller

And a woman spoke, saying,
"Tell us of Pain."
And he said,
"Your pain is the breaking of the shell
that encloses your understanding."

—Kahlil Gibran

The more the marble wastes, the more the statue grows.

—Michelangelo

By probing our own tragic dimension for its deeper story,
as well as raising it to a mythic level,
our wounding becomes the vehicle for grace
and we become spiritually charged
and able to live a larger and nobler life.

—Jean Houston

When life throws you a curve, it's to teach you how to bend.

—Anonymous

> If you would not have affliction visit you twice,
> listen at once to what it teaches.
>
> —*James Burgh*

Neurotics cannot seem to move beyond their story to broader contexts and deeper formulations. Your work is clear. It is not to change the story, for this is to deny it; it is, rather, to expand and deepen the story, thus releasing the energy bound within it.

> —*Jean Houston*

> The stars receive their brightness from the surrounding dark.
>
> —*Dante Alighieri*

> Suffering is a revelation.
> One discovers things one never discovered before.
>
> —*Oscar Wilde*

Soulmaking requires that you die to one story to be reborn to a large one. A renaissance, a rebirth, occurs not just because there is a rising of ancient and archetypal symbols. A renaissance happens because the soul is breached. In this wounding, the psyche is opened up and new questions begin to be asked about who we are in our depths.

> —*Jean Houston*

> Behold, I will send my messenger.
>
> —*Malachi 3:1*

Chapter 6: Sacred and Profane Wounds

Never does a man know the force that is in him
till some mighty affection or grief has humanized the soul.

—Frederick W. Robertson

As soon as suffering becomes acute enough,
one goes forward.

—Herman Hesse

A crisis is an attempt of nature, of the natural,
cosmic lawfulness of the universe, to effect change....
It tears and breaks up, which is momentarily painful,
but transformation is unthinkable without it.

—Eva Pierrakos

A larger story is revealed by the wounding....
The wounding becomes sacred when we are willing to release
our old stories and to become the vehicles through which
the new story may emerge into time....
Wounding opens the doors of our sensibility to a larger reality....

—Jean Houston

Go find the gem hidden in your depths!

—Jalaluddin Rumi

Friction polishes.

—Family member

Of course, there is no mind without restlessness;
restlessness is the very nature of the mind.

—Vasishtha

We have been tyrannized by the local,
historical psychological story.
While there is nothing wrong with this story,
which carries its own level of truth,
as the only story it is extremely limited, limiting, and isolating.

—Jean Houston

Betrayal of all the woundings that may be suffered by the soul can be the greatest agent of the sacred. This wound has always had an awful and luminous quality surrounding it. It marks the end of primal, unconscious trust, and forces upon us those terrible conditions that accompany the taking of the next step.

—Jean Houston

You do not get over a sacred wound.
You are transformed by it.

—Lois Gold

The needle that pierces
may carry a thread that binds us to heaven.

—James Hastings

Let's take the example of getting jilted…. How does the Soul view such historical events? Contrary to the way the Ego interprets those losses—identifying oneself as the "jilt-ee," the wronged party—the Soul sees a larger dance in motion. Looking back at such painful episodes from this consciousness, we may see that what appeared to be losses in fact led us to happier outcomes. Each of the Ego's "failures" has contributed to making us who we are now. Without meaning to sound saccharine: each step we take in our learning is, from the Soul's point of view, a blessing.

—*Ram Dass*

We are healed of a suffering only by experiencing it to the full.

—*Marcel Proust*

Experience everybody (or everything) in your life as either a teacher or a lover.

—*Ken Keyes, Jr.*

Great works are performed not by strength, but perseverance.

—*Samuel Johnson*

When symptoms persist and illness becomes chronic, we often find fault with the victim; we call it a lack of will power, a desire for attention, an unwillingness to work or change, rather than question the hidden assumption that is within our power as human beings to overcome sickness and, in fact, it is our job to do so.

—*Kat Duff*

Last night as I lay sleeping, I dreamt
O, marvelous error—
That there was a beehive here inside my heart
And the golden bees were making white combs
And sweet honey from all my failures.

—*Antonio Machado*

When we look at the shifts in our physical state
from a Soul perspective, the difference is remarkable:
instead of bemoaning the loss of who we were,
we marvel at who we are becoming.

—*Ram Dass*

Sweet are the uses of adversity, which like the toad,
ugly and venomous, wears yet a precious jewel in his head.

—*William Shakespeare*

Adversity has the effect of eliciting talents
which in prosperous circumstances would have lain dormant.

—*Horace*

Sacred psychology is the process and practice of soulmaking; and soulmaking, as you may have discovered, is not necessarily a happy thing.... As seed making begins with the wounding of the ovum by the sperm, so does soulmaking begin with the wounding of the psyche by the Larger Story.

—*Jean Houston*

Chapter 6: Sacred and Profane Wounds

> Bad times have scientific value.
> These are occasions a good learner would not miss.
> —*Ralph Waldo Emerson*

> It's not what you look at; it's what you see.
> —*Talmud*

> But tragedy carries a gift in its other hand
> and someday you will see this.
> —*Lois Gold*

> All wounds hurt.
> Some just make more sense than others do.
> These can propel us forward to our destiny.
> —*A man in recovery who had OCD for as long as he can remember*

> A life-shattering circumstance
> that invites us to be all we can be
> is a modern-day sacred wound.
> —*Herb Gravitz*

> Few men during their lifetime come anywhere near
> exhausting the resources dwelling within them.
> There are deep wells of strength that are never used.
> —*Richard E. Byrd*

In no way is suffering necessary to find meaning.
I only insist that meaning is possible even in spite of suffering.

—*Viktor Frankl*

—⚎—

Everything can be taken from a man but one thing:
the last of the human freedoms—
to choose one's attitude in any given set of circumstances,
to choose one's own way.

—*Viktor Frankl*

—⚎—

Composing a life involves a continual reimaging
of the future and reinterpretation of the past
to give meaning to the present.

—*Mary Catherine Bateson*

—⚎—

When I dare to be powerful—
to use my strength in the service of my vision—
then it becomes less and less important whether I am afraid.

—*André Lorde*

—⚎—

Only a life lived in a certain spirit is worthwhile. It is a remarkable fact that a life lived entirely from the ego [a profane wound] usually strikes not only the person himself, but observers also, as being dull.

—*Carl G. Jung*

—⚎—

Chapter 6: Sacred and Profane Wounds

I proceeded with the question [in a group meeting to a woman who lost her child and couldn't understand why this tragedy happened to her] whether an ape which was being used to develop polimyelitis serum, and for this reason punctured again and again, would ever be able to grasp the meaning of its suffering. Unanimously, the group replied that of course it would not; with its limited intelligence, it could not enter into the world of man, i.e., the only world in which the meaning of its suffering would be understandable. Then I pushed forward with the following question: "And what about man? Are you sure that the human world is a terminal point in the evolution of the cosmos? Is it not conceivable that there is still another dimension, a world beyond man's world; a world in which the question of an ultimate meaning of human suffering would find an answer?"

—*Viktor Frankl*

Freud once explained that when one looks at a crystal, the place where that crystal is broken is the place that most clearly reveals its structure. We can discover its essence by examining where it is cracked. In the same way, our own wounds can be vehicles for exploring our essential nature, revealing the deepest textures of our heart and soul, if only we will sit with them, open ourselves to the pain, and allow ourselves to be taught, without holding back, without blame.

—*Rev. Wayne Muller*

Life never presents us with anything
which may not be looked upon as a fresh starting point,
no less than as a termination.

—*André Gide*

The whole life of the individual is nothing but the process of giving birth to himself; indeed, we should be fully born, when we die, although it is the tragic fate of most individuals to die before they are born.

—Erich Fromm

―⚜―

Be witness to it, rather than a reactor to it.

—Gurudev (Yogi Amrit Desai)

―⚜―

The passage of the mythological hero may be from one geographical place to another, but fundamentally it is inward—into the depths where obscure resistances are overcome, and long-lost, forgotten powers are revivified, to be made available for the transfiguration of the world.

—Joseph Campbell

―⚜―

Life is a tragedy when seen in close-up
but a comedy in longshot.

—Charlie Chaplin

―⚜―

It takes one a long time to become young.

—Pablo Picasso

―⚜―

I have walked through the valley of the shadow of death—
and I have come out, not unscathed but undaunted.

—Mother of a son with OCD

―⚜―

Chapter 6: Sacred and Profane Wounds

> Life does not accommodate you, it shatters you....
> Every seed destroys its container
> or lest there would be no fruition.
>
> —*Florida Scott-Maxwell*

But lives, like plants, grow from rich mulch of decayed dreams and abortive efforts, whose effect on future growth is not duplicated by the logical 1-2-3 methods that we endorse in the advice we offer others.

> —*William Bridges*

> Decisions are made on the basis of evidence and logic,
> but choices are always an act of will.
>
> —*William Bridges*

> A profane wound leaves one feeling victimized,
> taken advantage of, put upon, and otherwise suffering
> from a meaningless encounter.
> It's all for naught! That is the real tragedy.
>
> —*Herb Gravitz*

It's not so much that we're afraid of change or so in love with the old ways, but it's that place in between that we fear....It's like being in between trapezes. It's Linus when his blanket is in the dryer. There's nothing to hold on to.

> —*Marilyn Ferguson*

The demon you swallow gives you its power.

—*Joseph Campbell*

All through history it is true that only by going through hell does one have any chance of reaching heaven. The journey through hell is a part of the journey that cannot be omitted—indeed, what one learns in hell is prerequisite to arriving at any good value thereafter. Homer has Odysseus visit the underworld, and there—and only there—can he get the knowledge that will enable him to get safely back to Ithaca. Virgil has Aeneas go into the netherworld and there talk to his father, in which discussion he got directions as to what to do and what not to do in the founding of the great city of Rome. How fitting it is that each of these gets a vital wisdom which is learned in the descent into hell!…The agony, the horror, the sadness, are a necessary prelude to self-realization and self-fulfilment.

—*Rollo May*

I have found that I am a lot tougher than I ever thought I could be. I have found confidence where I thought there was none. If I hadn't been pushed, and I mean I went dragging and kicking, pushing and screaming, I wouldn't have ever done it. I now smell the roses. I have started a garden, because I can pretty much control that. And I take my needs and myself a lot more seriously than I ever would have. It's no bowl of cherries, but it's no longer a can of worms either. It's been a tough way to learn!

—*Wife of a sufferer with OCD*

Emotion is the chief source of all becoming conscious. There can be no transformation of darkness into light… without emotion.

—*Carl Jung*

At that point I realized that I had been dealing with a very "refined" sort of grace in the past—the loving kind of grace, the grace of the good things that kept happening to me. "Fierce grace" means I've now been given a fully rounded understanding of grace. Now I have a full view of what grace is all about.

—Ram Dass

—⚏—

When there is no longer a cyclone, there is no longer an eye. So the storms, crises and sufferings of life are a way of finding the eye. When everything is going our way we do not see the eye and feel no need to look for it. But when everything is going against us, then we find the eye.

—Bernadette Roberts

—⚏—

Shortly thereafter, I began to leave my former identity, my Richard Alpert-ness, behind to embark upon a journey of becoming Ram Dass, or Servant of God—a journey that continues to this day. Looking back it is clear to me that the despair I experienced [from the stroke he had which essentially crippled his body] was a prerequisite to what came next. The negative thing, the depression, pushed me to find something. The positive thing, the spiritual growth, pulled me out of the depression. I have witnessed similar cycles among friends on the path to consciousness, when they spiral into deep depressions that prove, in time, to be preparation for something else.

—Ram Dass

—⚏—

I don't know what your destiny will be, but one thing I know: the only ones among you who will be really happy are those who have sought and found how to serve.

—Albert Schweitzer

—⚏—

When we set our sights on a higher meaning, we automatically cast ourselves in the role of a dweller at the threshold, an initiate in a Great Story. We are not powerless, trapped or worthless. We are passing through the fire on the way to a purification of sufficient value that our suffering becomes worthwhile when weighted against it.

—*Joan Borysenko*

The stroke was Maharjji's
[one of Ram Dass' beloved gurus]
lightning bolt to jolt me into a new place in my consciousness.
The ferocity of the method tested my faith,
but in the end my faith held.

—*Ram Dass*

What was changed through the stroke was my attachment to the Ego. The stroke was unbearable to the Ego, and so it pushed me into the Soul level also, because when you 'bear the unbearable,' something within you dies. My identity flipped over and I said, 'So that's who I am—I'm a Soul!' I ended up where looking at the world from the Soul level is my ordinary, everyday state—not an occasional experience, with psychedelics or for some other reason, but my everyday reality. And that's grace. That's almost the definition of grace.

—*Ram Dass*

I have made my world and it is a much better world
than I ever saw outside.

—*Louise Nevelson*

Chapter 6: Sacred and Profane Wounds

> Truly, it is in the darkness that one finds the light,
> so when we are in sorrow, then this light is nearest of all to us.
>
> —*Meister Eckhart*

Tragedy brings forward the need to create meaning—to tell new stories—that can reweave the frayed ends of life into a coherent whole. Our ability to tell these stories is positively linked with recovery….

—*Joan Borysenko*

> Man's main concern is not to gain pleasure or to avoid pain
> but rather to see a meaning in his life.
> That is why man is even ready to suffer, on the condition,
> to be sure, that his suffering has a meaning.
>
> —*Viktor Frankl*

When Bill [Bill Wilson, the co-founder of Alcoholics Anonymous] asked [Father Ed Dowling, a Jesuit priest, who visited Bill when he was in the midst of a "dry drunk" just before AA was to emerge on the national scene in the early 1940s] if there was never to be any satisfaction, the old man snapped back, "Never. Never any." There was only a kind of divine dissatisfaction that would keep him going, reaching out always.

—*Robert Thomsen*

> Grief begins with a terrible and lonely loss.
> Grief changes you but it is not destroying you.
> Grief is a powerful teacher.
>
> —*Rabbi Earl A. Grollman*

My barn having burned to the ground,
I can now see the moon.

—*Japanese folk saying*

My belief is that health and sickness are complementary opposites, that we cannot have one without the other, any more than good and evil can stand alone. The challenge is to use sickness as an opportunity for transformation.

—*Andrew Weil*

Teach us to number our days
that we may acquire a heart of wisdom.

—*Psalm 90:12*

Human life is not freedom from adverse conditions,
but freedom to take a stand on adversity.
To live is to suffer.
To survive is to find meaning in suffering.

—*Viktor Frankl*

Big success is not built on success.
It's built on adversity, failure, and frustration,
sometimes catastrophe,
and the way we deal with it and turn it around.

—*Sumner Redstone*

> Since we cannot change reality,
> let us change the eyes which see reality.
>
> —Nikos Kazantzakis

To understand things we must have been once in them and then have come out of them; so that first there must be captivity and then deliverance, illusion followed by disillusion, enthusiasm by disappointment. He who is still under the spell and he who has never felt the spell are equally incompetent.

> —Amiel

> Within us all there are wells of thought
> and dynamos of energy
> which are not suspected until emergencies arise.
>
> —Thomas J. Watson, Sr.

> No one is beat till he quits
> No one is through till he stops
> No matter how hard failure hits
> No matter how often he drops.
> A man's not dead till he lies
> In the dust and refuses to rise.
> Fate can slam him, and bang him around
> And batter his frame till he's sore.
> But no one can say that he's downed,
> While he bobs up serenely for more.
> A man's not dead till he dies
> Nor beat till no longer he tries.
>
> —Edgar A. Guest

> And the day came when the risk to remain tight in a bud
> was more painful than the risk it took to blossom.
> —*Anaïs Nin*

> The world breaks everyone
> and afterward many are strong at the broken places.
> —*Ernest Hemingway*

> Should you shield the canyons from the windstorms,
> you would never see the beauty of their carvings.
> —*Elisabeth Kübler-Ross*

> Beauty can come out of pain. But that doesn't make pain beautiful.
> —*Ashleigh Brilliant*

There is a constant theme of triumph over adversity as a sacred path throughout history. Triumph is not a matter of mind over matter, it is not a matter of willpower, and it is not simply positive thinking. Rather, it is the age-old alchemical process of turning the poisonous lead of one's horrific experience into the shining gold of our destiny to manifest our most sacred self.

Not everyone, however, chooses to accept the "call" for such a hallowed journey. When the call is refused, the result is always the same: a disaster of some major proportion for the individual. For refusal of the call is a betrayal of the self. Thus, there are always two great betrayals with illness, addiction, or other trauma. The first betrayal comes about from the circumstance. It may be faulty genetics, which predisposes the person to inherit something negative or horrific. It may be a poisonous environment, whether parental or societal. Such a betrayal, however, need not end in calamity or disaster.

As bad and as harmful as this type of external betrayal can be, however, it pales in comparison to the second betrayal. The worst betrayal of all occurs when the person betrays himself or herself. This self-betrayal unfolds as the person refuses to become what he can be by cheating himself with excuses and rationalizations. Such behaviors always lead to what one of the greatest evolutionary thinkers, Carl Jung, calls "inauthentic suffering"—an endless suffering that has no beginning, middle, or end and a suffering which offers a dull, boring, meaningless existence punctuated by cynicism and apathy.

For the person who dares to choose triumph, there is an alternative. This passage always involves moving through our "dark night—indeed our dark nights—of the soul." As noted mythologist Joseph Campbell stated: "The labyrinth is thoroughly known. We have only to follow the thread of the hero path, and where we had thought to find an abomination, we shall find a god. And where we had thought to slay another, we shall slay ourselves. Where we had thought to travel outward, we will come to the center of our existence. And where we had thought to be alone, we will be with all the world."

Betrayal from a mythic perspective opens a whole new vista by enlarging our stories and making the betrayal a route to discovery. Rather than a person, an event, or a circumstance that condemns one to suffering and pain, betrayal can be one of the greatest agents of the sacred. It is the end of our unconsciousness and naiveté. We must learn discernment and it can invite us to take the next step in our own growth and evolution.

It is this alternative path that we now address.

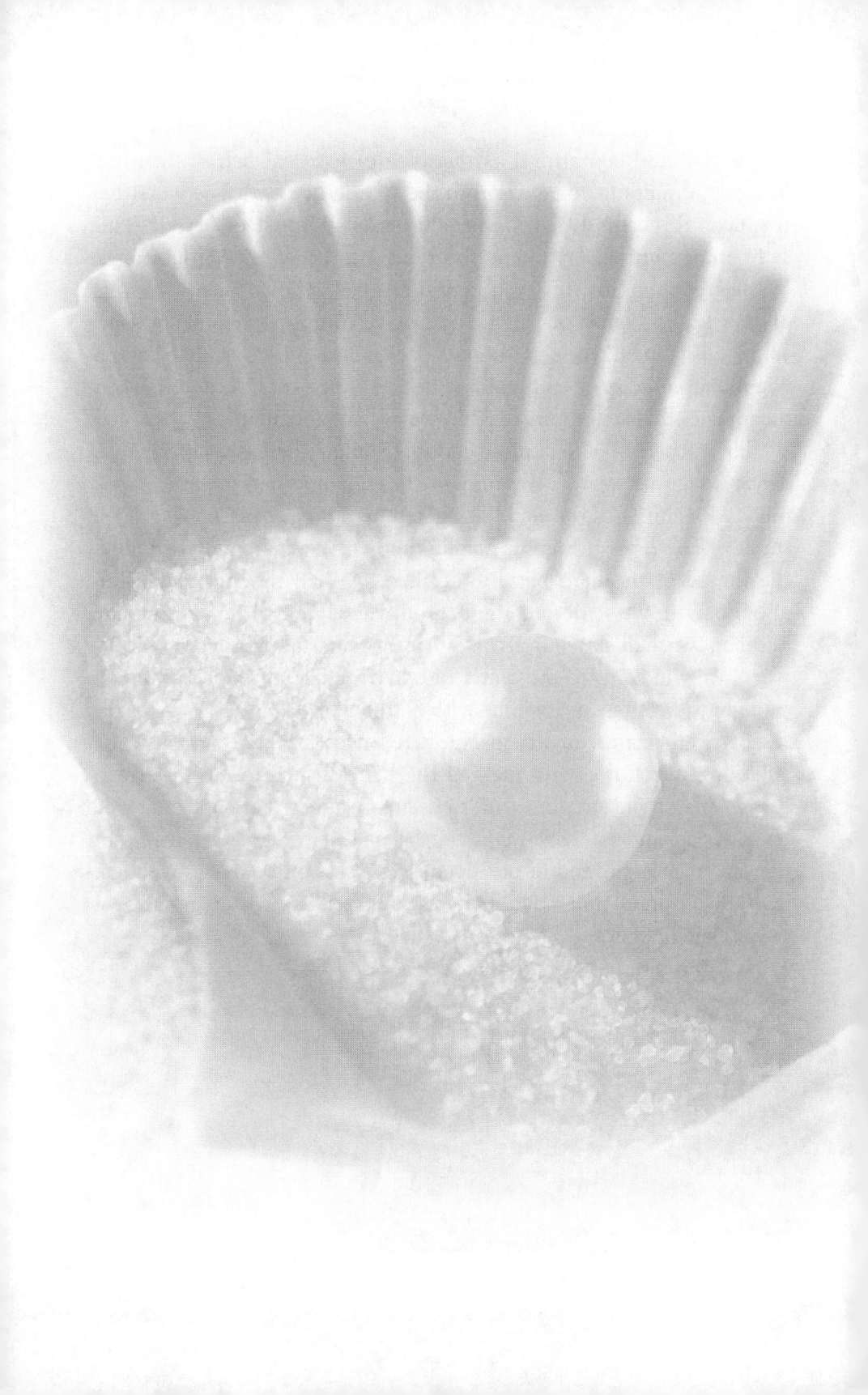

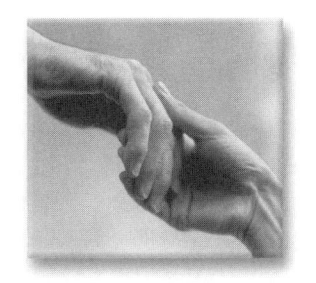

CHAPTER 7

The Journey

Every wound is the occasion for a journey, an odyssey no less dangerous or important than our ancestors undertook thousands of years ago to save the realm. The more gaping the wound, the greater the journey will be. Seldom easy or short, the path is always fraught with danger and opportunity. In fact, the occasion of the journey is typically a crisis. Recall that crisis is a word derived from the two Chinese symbols, danger and opportunity. Crises are the junction between danger and opportunity.

All members of the family under the influence of one of life's major wounds are exposed to this crossroads. If we are fortunate—or if we can surrender to the grace that accompanies life's great wounds—we will find someone or something to guide us through. Luke, the hero of the movie *Star Wars*, had Yoda. Like Luke, we find that our guide can come in many forms—a teacher, a friend, a therapist, a word, or words that heal.

Heroism and adversity are inexorably linked on every great journey. As the great writer F. Scott Fitzgerald wrote: "Show me a hero and I'll show you a tragedy." And like the heroes who have come before us and have accepted, however reluctantly, the journey, we can go forth on a divine journey described by the sages from all of time.

It is this route from tragedy to hero that is a universal journey. It is often described as consisting of three main stages. The first stage is "Separation." We leave that which has been familiar and comfortable. In mythological terms, the realm is under siege—usually by a monster such as a dragon—and a call is made for someone, the "hero" or "heroine," to leave home to do battle.

For family members the stage of separation starts with the onset of the illness, addiction, trauma, or other major life circumstance that may require a life very different than the person once knew. This initial stage removes us from the familiar and thrusts us into a situation that is unknown and frightening, such as a hospital, the mental health system, or to the brink of emotional and financial disaster. In this new situation, the rules are not known or poorly understood. The roles change, too, as we take on different functions and responsibilities. Spouses can become parents, parents can become children, even children can become parents.

This launches the second stage, or the "Initiation." In this stage we endure major trials that test our strength and courage. We are usually thrust into the darkness where we must do battle with our demons, face our monsters, and dispel the falsehoods and misunderstandings of a lifetime. A frightening time, often scarcely imaginable, it is full of doubt, confusion, and wonder.

For family members, this stage involves learning about the adversity, dealing with the false beliefs surrounding it, as well as dealing with their own possible feelings of fear and shame. All members of the family face this stage. Each must meet his or her demons. Like the primary sufferer, secondary sufferers have their own issues as well as their own descent and initiation into another life.

If we survive this part of the journey, we enter the third stage, or the "Return." Having left the familiar and fought our devils from within and without, we return home with the gifts that we have learned and share them with others. Unfortunately, it almost always happens that on the way home we get attacked. Home is thus not an easy journey itself. We are also not always greeted with open arms when we arrive.

Chapter 7: The Journey

The mythological hero, Odysseus, who conceived the brilliant idea of the Trojan Horse, which ended the war with Troy, took ten years to return home, only to find his home overrun with enemies. But because of all that he had learned on the way back, he was able to defeat them and triumph once again.

Many get discouraged by the length of time it takes to make the journey. When commenting on the length of time the journey can take, one family member said: "Yes, it takes a long time to recover—maybe three to five years. But three to five years will pass no matter what. You might as well have something to show for your time."

Let's look closer at what may be the most important journey any of us will take. We'll see its twists and turns, its ups and downs.

Toto, I have a feeling we're not in Kansas anymore.
—*Dorothy in the* Wizard of Oz

The journey of a thousand miles begins with the first step.
—*Lao Tsu*

There is only one journey. Going inside yourself.
—*Rainer Maria Rilke*

The trip becomes a journey after you have lost your luggage.
—*Anonymous*

Most heroic journeys involve going through a dark place—
through mountain caverns, the underworld,
or labyrinthine passages to emerge, finally, into the light.

—*Jean Shinoda Bolen*

The limbo—which lasted for twelve timeless days—started as torment, but turned into patience; started as hell, but became a purgatorial dark night; humbled me, horribly, took away hope, but then sweetly-gently, returned it to me thousandfold, transformed.

—*Oliver Sacks*

You work on yourself first. That is our only salvation.
We are the only one we can change.
No matter how John (her ill son) behaves,
we still must have our life.

—*Family member*

Impossible is not in my dictionary.

—*Napoleon*

Our life evokes our character.
You find out more about yourself as you go on.
That's why it's good to be able to put yourself in situations
that will evoke your higher nature
rather than your lower.

—*Joseph Campbell*

> As you go the way of life, you will see a great chasm.
> Jump. It is not as wide as you think.
>
> —From a Native American initiation rite

Creation myths are pervaded with a sense of the doom that is continually recalling all created shapes to the imperishable out of which they first emerged. The forms go forth powerfully, but inevitably reach their apogee, break, and return. Mythology, in this sense, is tragic in its view. But in the sense that it places our true being not in the forms that shatter but in the imperishable out of which they again immediately bubble forth, mythological is eminently unmagical. Indeed, where the mythological mood prevails, tragedy is impossible.

—Joseph Campbell

> Journeys bring power and love into you.
>
> —Jalaluddin Rumi

Now, as a person faced with serious illness.... I'd discovered that with a slight shift in perception, my illness could also become a journey of self-discovery. Having accepted the current realities of my life, I found, as many others have, that choosing to make this shift could lead to a sense of wholeness that makes life better, whether the disease gets better or not. I believe there are really no real catastrophes or disasters. There is only our interpretation of events, and how we choose to interpret them helps determine how we act toward them.

—Linda Noble Topf

The world is not to be put in order, the world is in order.
It is for us to put ourselves in unison with this order.

—Henry Miller

It is no easier, just more urgent when you are near death.

—Family member

Happiness is mostly a by-product
of doing what makes us feel fulfilled.

—Benjamin Spock

Happiness makes up in height
for what it lacks in length.

—Robert Frost

Happiness is not a state to arrive at,
but a manner of traveling.

—Margaret Lee Runbeck

Five senses; an incurably abstract intellect; a haphazardly selective memory; a set of preconceptions and assumptions so numerous that I can never examine more than a minority of them—never become even conscious of them all. How much of total reality can such an apparatus let through?

—C. S. Lewis

Chapter 7: The Journey

If you want happiness for a lifetime,
help the next generation.

—*Chinese proverb*

Courage is almost a contradiction in terms.
It means a strong desire to live
taking the form of a readiness to die.

—*G. K. Chesterton*

Only in growth, reform, and change
(paradoxically enough)
is true security to be found.

—*Anne Morrow Lindbergh*

Only a baby who is wet likes a change.

—*Anonymous*

Life shrinks or expands in proportion to one's courage.

—*Anaïs Nin*

Courage is doing what you're afraid to do.
There can be no courage unless you're scared.

—*Eddie Rickenbacker*

All adventures, especially into new territory, are scary.
—*Sally Ride*

None but a coward dares to boast
that he has never known fear.
—*Marshal Ferdinand Foch*

What counts is not necessarily the size of the dog in the fight—
it's the size of the fight in the dog.
—*Dwight David Eisenhower*

The question is not whether you're frightened or not, but whether you or the fear is in control. If you say, "I won't be frightened," and then you experience fear, most likely you'll succumb to it, because you're paying attention to it. The correct thing to tell yourself is, "If I do get frightened, I will stay in command."
—*Herbert Fensterheim*

The wind and the waves are always on the side
of the ablest navigators.
—*Edward Gibbon*

We must face what we fear;
that is the case of the core of the restoration of health.
—*Max Lerner*

Chapter 7: The Journey

> Whether you think you can or think you can't,
> you're right.
>
> —Henry Ford

> Excellence happens when high purpose
> and intense pragmatism meet.
>
> —Tom Peters

What is a hero? I remember the glib response I repeated so many times. My answer was that a hero is someone who commits a courageous action without considering the consequences—a soldier who crawls out of a foxhole to drag an injured buddy to safety. And I also meant individuals who are slightly larger than life: Houdini and Lindbergh, John Wayne, JFK, and Joe DiMaggio. Now my definition is completely different. I think a hero is an ordinary individual who finds the strength to persevere and endure in spite of overwhelming obstacles....

—Christopher Reeve

> The hero is the man or woman
> who has been able to battle past his personal
> and local historical limitations
> to the generally valid,
> normally human forms.
>
> —Joseph Campbell

> To believe in the heroic makes heroes.
>
> —Benjamin Disraeli

The recipe for well-being, then, requires neither positive nor negative thinking alone, but a mix of ample optimism to provide hope, a dash of pessimism to prevent complacency, and enough realism to discriminate those things we can control from those we cannot.

—*Reinhold Niebuhr*

Heroes are just common people extended to remarkable limits.

—*Family member*

And in truth, grief is a great teacher when it sends us back to serve and bless the living.... Thus, even when they are gone, the departed are with us, moving us to live as, in their higher moments, they themselves wished to live. We remember them now; they live in our hearts; they are an abiding blessing.

—*Jewish Kiddush*

Yard by yard, it's just too hard
Inch by inch, it's a cinch.

—*Anonymous*

A calm sea never makes a good mariner.

—*Old sailor's proverb*

It does not matter how slowly you go
as long as you do not stop.

—*Confucius*

An adventure is only an inconvenience,
rightly considered.

—*G. K. Chesterton*

When you're on a journey,
and the end keeps getting further and further away,
then you realize the real end is the journey.

—*Karlfried Graf Durkheim*

Every noble work is at first impossible.

—*Thomas Carlyle*

There is no way of seeing things without first taking leave of them.

—*Antonio Machado*

Justice without force is powerless;
force without justice is tyrannical.

—*Blaise Pascal*

It is better to protest than to accept injustice.

—*Rosa Parks*

A man cannot be comfortable without his own approval.

—*Mark Twain*

Grant that we may not so much seek to be understood
as to understand.

—*St. Francis of Assisi*

I long to accomplish a great and noble task,
but it is my chief duty to accomplish small tasks
as if they were great and noble.

—*Helen Keller*

There is no growth except in the fulfilment of obligations.

—*Antoine de Saint-Exupéry*

If a sense of duty tortures a man,
it also enables him to achieve prodigiously.

—*H. L. Mencken*

Become a possibilitarian.
No matter how dark things seem to be or actually are,
raise your sights and see the possibilities—
always see them,
for they're always there.

—*Norman Vincent Peale*

The greatest discovery of my generation is that a human being can alter his life by altering his attitudes of mind.

—*William James*

No man can always be right. So the struggle is to do one's best; to keep the brain and conscience clear; never to be swayed by unworthy motives or inconsequential reasons, but to strive to unearth the basic factors involved and then do one's duty.

—*Dwight David Eisenhower*

—∞—

Repetition is the key to mastery.

—*Herb Gravitz*

—∞—

There are no shortcuts to any place worth going.

—*Beverly Sills*

—∞—

To keep a lamp burning, we have to keep putting oil in it.

—*Mother Teresa*

—∞—

If we are facing in the right direction,
all we have to do is keep on walking.

—*Buddhist expression*

—∞—

Boys, there ain't no free lunches in this country. And don't go spending your whole life commiserating that you got the raw deals. You've got to say, "I think that if I keep working at this and want it bad enough I can have it." It's called perseverance.

—*Lee Iacocca*

—∞—

Work is love made visible.
—*Kahlil Gibran*

The harder you work, the luckier you get.
—*Gary Player*

Man's highest merit always is, as much as possible, to rule external circumstances and as little as possible to let himself be ruled by them.
—*Goethe*

Seriousness is the only refuge of the shallow.
—*Oscar Wilde*

We shall not flag or fail. We shall go on to the end. We shall fight in France, we shall fight on the seas and oceans, we shall fight with growing confidence and growing strength in the air. We shall defend our island, whatever the cost may be. We shall fight on the beaches, we shall fight on the landing grounds, we shall fight in the fields and in the streets, we shall fight in the hills; we shall never surrender.
—*Winston Churchill*

Do not be too timid and squeamish about your actions. All life is an experiment.
—*Ralph Waldo Emerson*

The first blow is half the battle.

—*Proverb*

When I thought I couldn't go on,
I forced myself to keep going.
My success is based on persistence,
not luck.

—*Estée Lauder*

Grieving is hard work—
work that tears at you in so many ways.
Grief taxes every part of you—
body, soul and spiritually.

—*Rabbi Earl A. Grollman*

Opportunity is missed by most people
because it is dressed in overalls and looks like work.

—*Thomas A. Edison*

No man drowns if he perseveres in praying to God—
and can swim.

—*Russian proverb*

Believe in miracles but be prepared for alternatives.

—*Old Jewish expression*

When you come to the end of your rope,
tie a knot and hang on.

—*Franklin D. Roosevelt*

Let's talk sense to the American people.
Let's tell them the truth,
that there are no gains without pains.

—*Adlai E. Stevenson*

Never give in! Never give in. Never, never, never. Never—
in anything great or small, large or petty—
never give in except to convictions of honor and good sense.

—*Winston Churchill*

Face the thing you fear the most
and it will certainly be the death of it.

—*Alfred Lord Tennyson*

My mother said to me,
"If you become a soldier you'll be a general;
if you become a monk you'll end up as the pope."
Instead, I became a painter and wound up as Picasso.

—*Pablo Picasso*

Pray to God, but keep rowing to the shore.

—*Russian proverb*

The healthy child experiences every emotion there is
to experience at least twice each day.

—*Malaysian proverb*

The game of life is a game of boomerangs.
Our thoughts, deeds, and words return to us sooner or later,
with astounding accuracy.

—*Florence Scovel Shin*

Human kindness has never weakened the stamina
or softened the fiber of a free people.
A nation does not have to be cruel to be tough.

—*Franklin D. Roosevelt*

We live very close together.
So, our prime purpose in this life is to help others.
And if you can't help them,
at least don't hurt them.

—*Dalai Lama*

To lose patience is to lose the battle.

—*Mahatma Gandhi*

I know God will not give me anything I can't handle.
I just wish that he didn't trust me so much.

—*Mother Teresa*

Turn your stumbling blocks into steppingstones.

—*Anonymous*

Failure is a detour, not a dead-end street.

—*Anonymous*

After a time of darkness comes the turning point.
The old is discarded and the new appears.
Persevere quietly on the path of inner truth.

—I Ching

As we say in the sewer,
if you're not prepared to go all the way,
don't put your boots on in the first place.

—*Television's Ed Norton on the old* Jackie Gleason Show

At first, dreams seem impossible,
then improbable,
then inevitable.

—*Christopher Reeve*

The journey itself is life;
therapy is no more than a major intervention along the way.

—*John Fortunato*

Chapter 7: The Journey

The Army.
Be all that you can be.
The greatest challenge of them all.
Yourself.

—*Advertisement*

We do not so much need the help of our friends
as the confidence of their help in need.

—*Epicurus*

Without a sense of proportion
there can be neither good taste nor genuine intelligence,
nor perhaps moral integrity.

—*Eric Hoffer*

I shall never believe that God plays dice with the world.

—*Albert Einstein*

Seven characteristics distinguish the wise: he does not speak in the presence of one wiser than himself, does not interrupt, is not hasty to answer, asks and answers the point, talks about first things first and about last things last, admits when he does not know, and acknowledges the truth.

—Talmud

There is nothing that will cure the senses but the soul, and nothing
that will cure the soul but the senses.

—Oscar Wilde

The future enters into us,
in order to transform itself in us,
long before it happens.

—Rainer Maria Rilke

So if your goal is to avoid pain and escape suffering, I would not advise you to seek higher levels of consciousness or spiritual evolution. First, you cannot achieve them without suffering, and second, insofar as you do achieve them, you are likely to be called upon to serve in ways more painful to you, or at least demanding of you, than you can possibly imagine.

—M. Scott Peck

Let's be our own heroes.

—Erin Brockovich

In every contest, there comes a moment that defines winning from losing. The true warrior understands and seizes that moment by giving an effort so intensive and so intuitive that it could only be called one from the heart.

—Pat Riley

After climbing a great hill, one only finds that there are many more hills to climb. I have taken a moment here to rest, to steal a view of the glorious vista that surrounds me, to look back on the distance I have come. But I can rest only for a moment, for with freedom comes responsibilities, and I dare not linger, for my long haul is not yet ended.

—*Nelson Mandela*

Popular tales represent the heroic action as physical; the higher religions show the deed to be moral.

—*Joseph Campbell*

For a long time it had seemed to me that life was about to begin—real life. But there was always some obstacle in the way. Something to be gotten through first, some unfinished business, time still to be served, a debt to be paid. Then life would begin. At last it dawned on me that these obstacles were my life.

—*Alfred D'Souza*

The amount you suffer in life is directly related to how much you are resisting that fact that things are the way they are.

—*Bill Harris*

The Rules for Being Human

1. You will receive a body. You may like it or hate it, but it will be yours for the entire period this time around.

2. You will learn lessons. You are enrolled in a full-time informal school called life. Each day in this school you will have the opportunity to learn lessons. You may like the lessons or think them irrelevant and stupid.

3. There are no mistakes, only lessons. Growth is a process of trial and error, experimentation. The "failed" experiments are as much a part of the process as the experiment that ultimately "works."

4. A lesson is repeated until learned. A lesson will be presented to you in various forms until you have learned it. When you have learned it, you can go on to the next lesson.

5. Learning lessons does not end. There is no part of life that does not contain its lessons. If you are alive there are lessons to be learned.

6. "There" is no better than "here." When your "there" has become a "here" you will simply obtain another "there" that will again look better than "here."

7. Others are merely mirrors of you. You cannot love or hate something about another person unless it reflects to you something you love or hate about yourself.

8. What you make of your life is up to you. You have all the tools and resources you need. What you do with them is up to you. The choice is yours.

9. Your answers lie inside you. The answer to life's questions lie inside you. All you need to do is look, listen, and trust.

10. This will often be forgotten, only to be remembered again.

—Cherie Carter-Scott

Look at every path closely and deliberately. Try it as many times as you think necessary. Then ask yourself and yourself alone one question. This question is one that only a very old man asks. My benefactor told me about it once when I was young and my blood was too vigorous for me to understand it. Now I do understand it. I will tell you what it is: Does this path have a heart? If it does, the path is good. If it doesn't it is of no use.

—*Carlos Castaneda*

The path to sainthood goes through adulthood.
There are no quick and easy shortcuts.

—*M. Scott Peck*

The road to wisdom is an obstacle course.

—*Tony Schwartz*

Such is the journey. It is described throughout all of history, in all cultures over the world, and by all its travelers everywhere. It is the journey of a lifetime; it is the journey for which we each are born—if we dare to take it.

In this book, you are invited to go on this most extraordinary journey. The path is well known, a reflection of the spirit that lives within us all. It is a story as old as time, a story of danger and opportunity, a momentous tale of the kingdom besieged.

All are called; only some make the quest. For both, nothing is ever the same. Everyone who lives under the influence of any major adversity is either on a journey of healing and triumph or one of sickness and defeat. Their choice, as we have seen in the last chapter, is to make it sacred or profane. Rather than one climactic journey, however, it is a subtle and extended journey, one that unfolds on a daily basis.

On this voyage, rather than the kingdom, it is the realm of the family that is at stake. On this odyssey, body and mind, soul and spirit, are in jeopardy. The outcome of the trials and tribulations of the journey can affect the welfare of every member of the family, as well as its future generations.

Just as in the old, great stories, a person is summoned, or presented with "the call," and asked to face the forces that threaten the realm of the family. Although the person is given an extraordinary feat to accomplish, he or she is typically quite ordinary, just like in the tales of all our great myths. This person is usually reluctant to accept the assignment, and may not believe that it can even be accomplished.

Our hero or heroine, as the person comes to be known in these tales, is no less a hero now than then. He or she goes forth, albeit with fear and trepidation, to fight the forces that threaten the realm, facing great, often extraordinary, adversities and overcoming enormous odds in order to triumph. As we have seen, along the way there are trials or tests that the person must pass in order to save the kingdom. At times, there are magicians, sorcerers, and guides along the way who may help in charting the territory, or who may try to block the path. After successfully confronting dragons and demons or whatever other mythical dilemmas, our hero now turns toward home.

The process of returning home is a unique part of the hero or heroine's journey, itself also fraught with danger and intrigue. For family members, this usually involves a process of "refamilying," a critical concept that we will explore in greater depth in a later chapter, in which there is a "return home."

But first, we understand that there are useful directions—attitudes, behaviors, and tools—that will make the journey possible. It is to these ways of accomplishing the journey that we now turn. Then we become practiced at what we must learn. There are many responses upon hearing about this journey, however, for the journey is never easy. But as one of my teachers once said: "Don't bite my finger; look where I'm pointing."

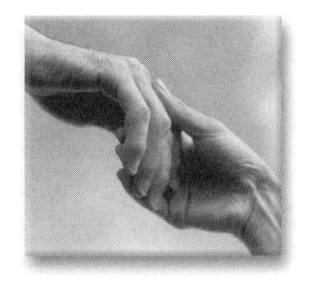

CHAPTER 8

The Method

How can we navigate the perilous path that is often in front of us? It is never an easy journey. Its waters are always uncharted. What tools do we need? What preparations are necessary? What attitudes will help? What will hinder us? Without a method, without tools for the encounter, we are more likely to be blown hither and yon, like a leaf in a raging wind.

Methods are a difficult term to define. They include so many different means. Are they a set of strategies, an arsenal of technological tools, special attitudes, or unique relationships? What is the best way to acquire them? Can words provide a container to hold all our sorrow, all our grief, all our wounding? Can words inspire us to go beyond what we ever thought was possible? If they couldn't, would they have stood the test of time?

Whatever we call them—learning strategies, coping skills, or the right attitudes and relationships—making lemonade out of life's lemons is the key to the transformational process. There are many guidelines to help. The wonderful thing about these guidelines being presented in metaphoric form, like in this book of healing, is that they affect each reader differently and in accord with her or his own unique personality.

Metaphors through aphorisms, proverbs, or precepts go to the very part of the brain that processes information rapidly and profoundly. They bypass the more conscious and critical parts of the brain, which operate under constraints such as "I can't."

Neither fantasy nor pipe dream, with the proper method(s), such as words that heal, we can triumph over almost anything! Life is replete with example after example of people who not only survive but also actually thrive in the midst of horrendous experiences. Somehow, the common denominator among these people is that they learn to construct powerful meanings for their circumstances.

> To know how to wonder and question
> is the first step of the mind toward discovery.
>
> —*Louis Pasteur*

Facts are neutral until human beings add their own meaning to those facts. People make their decisions based on what the facts mean to them, not on the facts themselves. The meaning they add to facts depends on their current story. People stick with their story even when presented with facts that don't fit. They simply interpret or discount the facts to fit their story. This is why facts are not terribly useful in influencing others. People don't need new facts—they need a new story.

—*Annette Simmons*

> Without perception of the unique meaning
> of his singular existence,
> a person would be numbed in difficult situations.
>
> —*Viktor Frankl*

Chapter 8: The Method

> This is what fools people:
> a man is always a teller of tales,
> he lives surrounded by his stories and the stories of others,
> he sees everything that happens to him through them;
> and he tries to live his own life as if he were telling a story.
>
> —*Jean-Paul Sartre*

> All sorrows can be borne if you put them into a story
> or tell a story about them.
>
> —*Isak Dinesen*

Family members' readiness to redefine the patient as different is critical to their ability to accommodate changes imposed by the illness.... When redefining is limited.... [They] do not experience any sense of personal growth from the experience: they simply endure it and wait for it to end.

—*Betty Davies*

> The lack of meaning in life
> is a soul-sickness whose full extent and full import
> our age has not as yet begun to comprehend.
>
> —*Carl G. Jung*

> God made man because he loves stories.
>
> —*Elie Wiesel*

We know everything we need to know to end the needless emotional suffering that many people currently experience.

—*Jack Canfield and Mark Victor Hansen*

Ask and it shall be given you;
Seek, and you shall find;
Knock, and it shall be opened to you.
For whoever asks, receives; and
He who seeks, finds; and to him who knocks,
the door is opened.

—*Jesus, in Matthew 7:7,8*

I wanted less to recover what I had had
than to discover what else I might become.

—*Arthur Frank*

The only place where success comes before work
is a dictionary.

—*Mark Twain*

You cannot make yourself feel something you do not feel,
but you can make yourself do right
in spite of your feelings.

—*Pearl Buck*

> There is nothing which persevering effort
> and unceasing and diligent care cannot overcome.
>
> —*Seneca*

> Until one is committed,
> there is hesitancy,
> the chance to draw back,
> always ineffectiveness....
> The moment one definitely commits oneself,
> then Providence moves, too.
> All sorts of things occur to help one
> that would never otherwise have occurred....
> Boldness has genius, power and magic in it.
> Begin it now....
>
> —*Goethe*

> There are four means of experiencing the pain of problems constructively that I call discipline: delaying of gratification, acceptance of responsibility, dedication to truth, and balancing.
>
> —*M. Scott Peck*

> We admitted we were powerless over alcohol
> [sex, money, obsessions and compulsions,
> and almost 250 other "problems"]—
> that our lives had become unmanageable.
>
> —*The first step of Alcoholics Anonymous
> and other Twelve-Step Programs*

Habit is overcome by habit.
—*Thomas à Kempis*

God gave burdens, and also shoulders.
—*Yiddish proverb*

The secret of a warrior is that he believes without believing.... To just believe would exonerate him from examining his situation. A warrior, whenever he has to involve himself with believing, does it as a choice.
—*Carlos Castaneda*

If God was patient with Job, I reasoned, he would be patient with me too. Besides, my anger was problem enough in itself, for I knew that anger can turn easily into bitterness. I did not want to exacerbate that problem by believing that God was so fragile that he could not absorb my anger [his mother, wife, and daughter were killed by a drunk driver in a car in which he was driving].
—*Gerald L. Sittser*

Hatred and bitterness can never cure the disease of fear;
only love can do that.
Hatred paralyzes life; love releases it.
Hatred confuses life. Love harmonizes it.
Hatred darkens life; love illuminates it.
—*Martin Luther King, Jr.*

Chapter 8: The Method

> Formula for longevity:
> Have a chronic illness and take good care of it.
>
> —*Oliver Wendell Holmes*

I doubt if any alcoholic ever wakes up, looks out the window, and says, "This would be a nice day to go for rehabilitation. I think I'll call the doctor." He may not see the gun, but some type of pressure—outside forces or his health—motivates him.

—*Thomas Fleming*

> We need four hugs a day for survival.
> We need eight hugs a day for maintenance.
> We need twelve hugs a day for growth.
>
> —*Virginia Satir*

> It isn't for the moment you are stuck that you need courage,
> but for the long uphill climb back to sanity
> and faith and security.
>
> —*Anne Morrow Lindbergh*

> Anxiety in human life is what squeaking and grinding
> are in machinery that is not oiled.
> In life, trust is the oil.
>
> —*Henry Ward Beecher*

Success isn't a result of spontaneous combustion.
You must set yourself on fire.

—Arnold Glascow

You don't always get what you ask for,
but you never get what you don't ask for...
unless it's contagious!

—Franklyn Broude

You miss 100 percent of the shots you never take.

—Wayne Gretzky

Great things are only possible with outrageous requests.

—Thea Alexander

To see things in the seed, that is genius.

—Lao Tzu

When we recognize where our power truly comes from,
we become blessed.

—Ben Vereen

You must be the change you wish to see in the world.

—Mahatma Gandhi

The sense of obligation to continue is present in all of us.
A duty to strive is the duty of us all.
I felt a call to that duty.

—Abraham Lincoln

They turn pain into a deeper understanding of themselves
and of what it means to be human.

—Mary Pipher

I had done an extraordinary thing
with no other tools than my own conviction.

—Erin Brockovich

The laughless people are the most dangerous.

—Robert Raines

Faith is not a cushion for me to fall back upon;
it is my working energy.

—Helen Keller

Faith makes all things possible.
Love makes all things easy.

—Rabbi Sidney Greenberg

God helps the brave.

—J. C. F. von Schiller

Encouragement is the oxygen of the soul.

—Anonymous

Without faith man becomes sterile, hopeless,
and afraid to the very core of his being.

—Erich Fromm

Courage is never to let your actions
be influenced by your fears.

—Arthur Koestler

Faith is the true force of life.

—Leo Tolstoy

Man who waits for roast duck to fly into mouth
must wait very, very, long time.

—Chinese Proverb

If you don't ask, you don't get.

—Mahatma Gandhi

> Do the thing you fear and the death of fear is certain.
> —*Ralph Waldo Emerson*

> First you jump off the cliff
> and you build your wings on the way down.
> —*Ray Bradbury*

> Action conquers fear.
> —*Peter Zarienga*

> If we wish to conquer undesirable emotional tendencies in ourselves, we must assiduously, and in the first instance cold-bloodedly, go through the outward motions of those contrary dispositions we prefer to cultivate.
> —*William James*

> Heaven ne'er helps the men who will not act.
> —*Sophocles*

> The first step is the hardest.
> —*Anonymous*

> I have become strong enough to forgive.
> —*Family member*

Do the thing you fear and keep on doing it…
that is the quickest and surest way ever yet discovered
to conquer fear.

—*Dale Carnegie*

If I continued to hate the illness,
I would be giving it more power than it deserves.
Forgiving is a way of banishing the illness from my soul.

—*Family member*

Such is the value of social occasions—calls, visits, dinners out:
They impel us to behave as if we were happy,
which in fact helps free us from our unhappiness.

—*David G. Myers*

My obligation is to do the right thing.
The rest is in God's hands.

—*Martin Luther King, Jr.*

Man must cease attributing his problems to his environment,
and learn again to exercise his will—
his personal responsibility in the realm of faith and morals.

—*Albert Schweitzer*

What cannot be altered must be borne, not blamed.

—*Thomas Fuller*

Laughter is the shortest distance between two people.
—*Victor Borge*

It is not miserable to be blind;
it is miserable to be incapable of enduring blindness.
—*John Milton*

Find what is divine, holy, or sacred for you.
Attend to it, worship it, in your own way.
—*Morrie Schwartz*

A certain excessiveness
seems a necessary element in all greatness.
—*Harvey Cushing*

Scientific studies have revealed that when we smile,
endorphins are released in the brain.
Smiling creates an instantaneous, safe,
and completely natural "high."
—*Elaine St. James*

Always bear in mind that our own resolution to success
is more important than any other one thing.
—*Abraham Lincoln*

I shall be telling this with a sigh
Somewhere ages and ages hence;
Two roads diverged in a wood, and I—
I took the one less traveled by,
And that has made all the difference.

—Robert Frost

You must do the thing you think you cannot do.

—Eleanor Roosevelt

Acceptance of what is truly happening is the first step to overcoming the consequences of misfortune.

—William James

The brain is like a muscle.
When we think well, we feel good.
Understanding is a kind of ecstasy.

—Carl Sagan

In the practice of tolerance, one's enemy is the best teacher.

—Dalai Lama

Deep in my heart I do believe
We shall overcome someday!

—Martin Luther King, Jr.

My folks were immigrants and they fell under the spell of the American legend that the streets were paved with gold. When Papa got here he found out three things: (1) The streets were not paved with gold; (2) The streets were not even paved; (3) He was supposed to do the paving.

—*Sam Levenson*

Love is the ability to extend one's self
for the purpose of nurturing one's own
or another's spiritual growth.

—*M. Scott Peck*

Students who sing or play an instrument score up to fifty-one points higher on the SATs than the national average. Music can strengthen your mind, unlock your creativity, and even heal your body.

—*Elaine St. James*

Courage in danger is half the battle.

—*Plautus*

Be grateful that you have been given the time to learn how to die.

—*Morrie Schwartz*

Have patience—everything is difficult before it is easy.

—*Saadi*

Grieving is the act of affirming or reconstructing a personal world of meaning that has been challenged by loss.... A narrative model is helpful in understanding this process of meaning reconstruction, which we regard as the central dynamic of grieving. If life is viewed as a story, then loss can be viewed as disrupting the continuity of the narrative. Like a novel that loses a central supporting character in a middle chapter, the life disrupted by bereavement forces its 'author' to envision far-reaching plot changes in order for the story to move forward in an intelligible fashion. Moreover, chronic and protracted losses may gradually erode the plot structure of the 'text' of one's biography, requiring continual revisions in the direction of one's life narrative, just at the point that we as authors have found a point of tenuous predictability. Constructing a way of bridging the past with a changing and uncertain future can be a major task, one that may require therapeutic support.

—Robert A. Neimeyer

A study of 12,238 men ages 35 to 57 found that, with other factors controlled, men who took annual vacations were 21 percent less likely to die during the 16-year study period than non-vacationers—and 32 percent less likely to die of coronary heart disease.

—Time *magazine*

Ninety percent of inspiration is perspiration.

—*Thomas Edison*

You can't wait for inspiration.
You have to go after it with a club.

—*Jack London*

> Seek Allah, but tether your camel first.
>
> —*Ancient proverb*

> A spoonful of honey will catch more flies
> than a gallon of vinegar.
>
> —*Ben Franklin*

> There is a certain criterion by which you can judge whether the thoughts you are thinking and the things you are doing are right for you. The criterion is: Have they brought you inner peace? If they have not, there is something wrong with them.
>
> —*Peace Pilgrim*

> When you shoot an arrow of truth,
> dip its point in honey.
>
> —*Arab proverb*

> Family members who seek and get help
> demonstrate and model effective coping and healing.
>
> —*Herb Gravitz*

> Commit yourself to a dream…. Nobody who tries to do something great but fails is a total failure. Why? Because he can always rest assured that he succeeded in life's most important battle—he defeated the fear of trying.
>
> —*Robert H. Schuller*

There is no such thing as great talent
without great willpower.

—Honoré de Balzac

When the going gets tough, the tough get going.

—Joseph P. Kennedy

An optimist sees an opportunity in every calamity;
a pessimist sees a calamity in every opportunity.

—Winston Churchill

When you pray for the potatoes, reach for the hoe.

—Alcoholics Anonymous saying

Big shots are only little shots who keep shooting.

—Dale Carnegie

The best way out is always through.

—Robert Frost

Do not seek to understand that you might have faith;
seek faith that you might understand.

—St. Augustine

The more we love our friends, the less we flatter them;
it is by excusing nothing that pure love shows itself.

—*Jean-Baptiste Molière*

And ye shall know the truth, and the truth shall make you free.

—*John 8:32*

The moral virtues are habits, and habits are formed by acts.

—*Robert M. Hutchins*

The most difficult thing in the world
is to know how to do a thing
and to watch someone else doing it wrong,
without commenting.

—*T. H. White*

Never let the fear of striking out get in your way.

—*Babe Ruth*

You can have anything in this world you want,
if you want it badly enough and you're willing to pay the price.

—*Mary Kay Ash*

Remember, a closed mouth gathers no foot.
—*Steve Post*

I can honestly say that I was never affected by the question of the success of an undertaking. If I felt it was the right thing to do, I was for it regardless of the possible outcome.
—*Golda Meir*

The eight grades of charity:
1. to give reluctantly
2. to give cheerfully but not adequately
3. to give cheerfully and adequately, but only after being asked
4. to give cheerfully, adequately, and of our own free will, but to put it in the recipient's hand in such a way as to make him feel less
5. to let the recipient know who the donor is, but not the reverse
6. to know who is receiving your charity but to remain anonymous to him
7. to have neither the donor nor the recipient be aware of the other's identity
8. to dispense with charity altogether, by enabling your fellow humans to have the wherewithal to earn their own living

—*Moses Maimonides*

Drown not thyself to save a drowning man.
—*Thomas Fuller*

Chapter 8: The Method

What value has compassion
that does not take its object in its arms?

—*Antoine de Saint-Exupéry*

If you want to lift yourself up,
lift up someone else.

—*Booker T. Washington*

Giving is the secret of a healthy life.
Not necessarily money,
but whatever a man has of encouragement
and sympathy and understanding.

—*John D. Rockefeller, Jr.*

Affection is created by habit, community of interests,
convenience, and the desire of companionship.
It is a comfort rather than an exhilaration.

—*W. Somerset Maugham*

You gotta look inside yourself.
You gotta look inside your inner self and find out who you are.

—*From the movie* **Analyze This**

Be aware that a halo has to fall only a few inches to be a noose.

—*Dan McKinnon*

Giving is the highest expression of potency.
—*Erich Fromm*

Teach us delight in simple things.
—*Rudyard Kipling*

The unfortunate need people who will be kind to them;
the prosperous need people to be kind to.
—*Aristotle*

Love cannot remain by itself—it has no meaning.
Love has to be put into action and that action is service.
—*Mother Teresa*

To be happy, drop the words *if only*
and substitute instead the words *next time*.
—*Smiley Blanton*

He that would eat the fruit must climb the tree.
—*James Kelly*

The foot of the farmer is the best manure of his land.
—*German proverb*

The whole idea of compassion is based on a keen awareness of the interdependence of all these living beings, which are all part of one another, and all involved in one another.

—*Thomas Merton*

Before you focus on finding the right person,
concentrate on being the right person.

—*Michael Levine*

To ensure time to think, reflect, and ponder, schedule meetings with yourself and honor them as you would an appointment with another.

—*Michael Levine*

Generally speaking,
the great achieve their greatness
by industry rather than by brilliance.

—*Bruce Barton*

The human body experiences a powerful gravitational pull in the direction of hope. That is why the patient's hopes are the physician's secret weapon. They are the hidden ingredients in any prescription.

—*Norman Cousins*

In Israel, in order to be a realist, you must believe in miracles.

—*David Ben-Gurion*

Someone once said to me, "Reverend Schuller, I hope you live to see all your dreams fulfilled." I replied, "I hope not, because if I live and all my dreams are fulfilled, I'm dead." It's the unfulfilled dreams that keep you alive.

—Robert Schuller

To travel hopefully is better than to arrive.

—Sir James Jeans

Hope is putting faith to work when doubting would be easier.

—Anonymous

Hope is wanting something so eagerly that—in spite of all the evidence that you're not going to get it—you go right on wanting it. And the remarkable thing about it is that this very act of hoping produces a kind of strength of its own.

—Norman Vincent Peale

Hope for the best, but prepare for the worst.

—English proverb

Everything that is done in the world is done by hope.

—Martin Luther King, Jr.

You've got to do your own growing,
no matter how tall your grandfather was.

—*Irish proverb*

Skepticism is the beginning of faith.

—*George Bernard Shaw*

Every human being is born without faith.
Faith comes only through the process of making decisions
to change before we can be sure it's the right move.

—*Robert Schuller*

We live by faith or we do not live at all. Either we venture—or we vegetate. If we venture, we do so by faith simply because we cannot know the end of anything at its beginning. We risk marriage on faith or we stay single. We prepare for a profession by faith or we give up before we start. By faith we move mountains of opposition or we are stopped by molehills.

—*Harold Walker*

The 4 C's:
We didn't cause it,
we can't control it,
we can't cure it,
but we can cope with it.

—*Al-Anon*

There are two sentences inscribed upon the Delphi oracle…
"Know thyself" and "Nothing too much"
and upon these all other precepts depend.

—Plutarch

Do not consider painful what is good for you.

—Euripides

If there is no wind, row.

—Proverb

Only the intelligent can understand what is obvious and what is concealed. Strength may be good or it may be evil. The same is true of weakness. The ideal is moderation.

—Chou-Tun-I

Great wisdom consists in not demanding too much
of human nature, and yet not altogether spoiling
it by indulgence.

—Lin Yutang

To believe in God is impossible—
not to believe in Him is absurd.

—Voltaire

Chapter 8: The Method

If men live decently
it is because discipline saves their very lives for them.

—*Sophocles*

I am not afraid of storms,
for I am learning how to sail my ship.

—*Louisa May Alcott*

As one goes through life one learns
that if you don't paddle your own canoe,
you don't move.

—*Katherine Hepburn*

A man's wisdom is most conspicuous
where he is able to distinguish among dangers
and make choice of the least.

—*Machiavelli*

I do not believe that sheer suffering teaches. If suffering alone taught, all the world would be wise, since everyone suffers. To suffering must be added mourning, understanding, patience, love, openness, and the willingness to remain vulnerable.

—*Anne Morrow Lindbergh*

Obstacles teach, not defeat.

—*Herb Gravitz*

There are no guarantees.
From the viewpoint of fear none are strong enough.
From the viewpoint of love none are necessary.
—*Emmanuel*

A miracle is a coincidence
in which God chooses to remain anonymous.
—*Gerald Jampolsky*

Don't wait for your ship to come; swim out to it.
—*Anonymous*

The great thing in this world is not so much where we are
but in which direction we are moving.
—*Oliver Wendell Holmes*

Wisdom consists not so much in knowing what to do
in the ultimate as in knowing what to do next.
—*Herbert Hoover*

Few things help an individual more
than to place responsibility upon him,
and to let him know that you trust him.
—*Booker T. Washington*

Do not seek to have everything that happens as you wish,
but wish for everything to happen as it actually does happen,
and your life will be serene.

—*Epictetus*

The U.S. Constitution doesn't guarantee happiness,
only the pursuit of it.
You have to catch up to it yourself.

—*Benjamin Franklin*

Bravery is the capacity to perform properly
even when scared half to death.

—*General Omar Bradley*

The important thing is this:
to be able at any moment to sacrifice
what we are for what we could become.

—*Charles DuBois*

Happiness depends upon ourselves.

—*Aristotle*

Courage is not the absence of fear,
but the willingness and ability to act despite one's fear.

—*Mark Twain*

When one's expectations are reduced to zero,
one really appreciates what one does have.

—Stephen Hawking

Fortitude is the marshal of thought,
the armor of the will,
and the fort of the reason.

—Francis Bacon

Power is ability to move from failure to failure
with enthusiasm.

—Winston Churchill

Love is energy.

—Marianne Williamson

Decisions are made on the basis of evidence and logic,
but choices are always an act of will.

—William Bridges

Let me not pray to be sheltered from dangers but to be fearless in facing them. Let me not pray for the stilling of my pain but for the heart to conquer it. Let me not crave in anxious fear to be saved but hope for the patience to win my freedom.

—Rabindranath Tagore

Only by contact with evil could I have learned to feel
by contrast the beauty of truth and love and goodness.
—*Helen Keller*

Fall seven times, stand up eight.
—*Japanese proverb*

When life gives you a lemon, make lemonade.
—*Anonymous*

The wishbone will never replace the backbone.
—*Will Henry*

Turn off your computer,
turn off your machine, and do it yourself,
follow your feelings, trust your feelings.
—*Ben Kenobi to Luke Skywalker in the climactic moment
of the last fight in the first* Star Wars *movie.*

A reverence for life is the antidote to addiction.
—*Charlotte Davis Kasl*

Courage is the thing. All goes if courage goes.
—*J. M. Barrie*

To gain that which is worth having,
it may be necessary to lose everything.

—Bernadette Devlin

This will remain the land of the free
only so long as it is the home of the brave.

—Elmer Davis

The world doesn't get better; you get better.

—Alcoholics Anonymous slogan

You can gain strength, courage, and confidence by every experience in which you really stop to look fear in the face.... You must do the thing which you think you cannot do.

—Eleanor Roosevelt

We can never discover new oceans
unless we have courage to lose sight of the shore.

—André Gide

A hero is no braver than an ordinary man,
but he is brave five minutes longer.

—Ralph Waldo Emerson

Chapter 8: The Method

It is not the critic who counts, not the man who points out how the strong man stumbled or where the doer of good deeds could have done better. The credit belongs to the man who is actually in the arena; whose face is marred by dust and sweat and blood; who strives valiantly; who errs and comes short again and again; who knows the great enthusiasms, the great devotions, and spends himself in a worthy cause; who at the best, knows in the end the triumph of high achievement; and who at the worst, if he fails, at least fails while daring greatly, so that his place shall never be with those cold and timid souls who know neither victory nor defeat.

—*Theodore Roosevelt*

Because of deep love, one is courageous.

—*Lao Tzu*

For some secondary survivors,
information about the effects of trauma on individuals
and relationships may be all that is necessary.

—*Charles R. Figley*

Taken together, the research on resilient individuals has increasingly pointed toward the importance of a systemic view. Worldwide studies of children of misfortune have found the most significant positive influence to be a close, caring relationship with a significant adult who believed in them and with whom they could identify, who acted as an advocate for them, and from whom they could gather strength to overcome their hardships.

—*Froma Walsh*

While troubles will come, they are always temporary—
nothing lasts forever.
Thus there is the famous legend that King Solomon,
the wisest man of all times,
had a ring inscribed with the words,
"This too will pass."

—*Rabbi Aryeh Kaplan*

Only by achieving a healthy balance
between the needs of self and those of others
can a secondary survivor offer support to a PTSD victim.

—*Charles R. Figley*

If I am not for myself, who will be for me?
If I am not for others, what am I?

—*Rabbi Hillel*

It is critical that all therapists who work with trauma victims and their families understand the parallel processes of individual and systemic stress reactions that may occur and remain present for years following a traumatic event.

—*Charles R. Figley*

I can solve a problem only when I say,
"this is my problem and it's up to me to solve it."

—*M. Scott Peck*

Chapter 8: The Method

> To one who waits all things reveal themselves,
> so long as you have the courage not to deny in the darkness
> what you have seen in the light.
> —*Coventry Patmore*

Family processes mediate the impact of stress on all members and their relationships.... The same stressors can lead to different outcomes, depending on how a family meets its challenges.
—*Froma Walsh*

> Families are blamed, not trained!
> —*A distraught parent*

I think it's a mistake to ever look for hope outside of one's self. One day the house smells of fresh bread, the next of smoke and blood. One day you faint because the gardener cut his finger off; within a week you're climbing over corpses of children bombed in a subway. What hope can there be if that is so? I tried to die near the end of the war. The same dream returned each night until I dared not to sleep and grew quite ill. I dreamed I had a child, and even in the dream I saw it was my life, and it was an idiot, and I ran away. But it always crept onto my lap again, clutched at my clothes. Until I thought, if I could kiss it, whatever in it was my own, perhaps I could sleep. And I bent to its broken face, and it was horrible...but I kissed it. I think one must finally take one's life in one's arms.
—*Arthur Miller*

When a man is willing and eager, the gods join in.
—Aeschylus

When I have forgiven myself and remembered who I am,
I will bless everyone and everything I see.
—A Course in Miracles

People who hold selective positive biases about stressful situations tend to do better than those who have a hard grasp of a reality that may be depressing, such as a life-threatening illness. These "positive illusions" sustain hope in the face of crisis, enabling such individuals to carry on their best efforts to overcome the odds.
—Froma Walsh

Hope…is neither passive waiting nor is it unrealistic forcing of circumstances that cannot occur. It is like the crouched tiger, which will jump only when the moment for jumping has come. To hope means to be ready at every moment for that which is not yet born, and yet not become desperate if there is no birth in our lifetime.
—Erich Fromm

By their openness, people dedicated to the truth live in the open, and through the exercise of their courage to live in the open, they become free from fear.
—M. Scott Peck

Chapter 8: The Method

The road to success is always under construction.

—*Anonymous*

The way you get meaning into your life is to devote yourself to loving others, devote yourself to your community around you, and devote yourself to creating something that gives you purpose and meaning.

—*Morrie Schwartz*

One ought every day at least to hear a little song,
read a good poem, see a fine picture,
and, if it were possible, to speak a few reasonable words.

—*Goethe*

I have learned that if I can just change my own part
in a situation, then other family members are much more likely
to change themselves.

—*Family member*

Discipline is the highest form of freedom.

—*Breck Costin*

Don't slow down; calm down!

—*Bumper sticker*

Included in this close fraternity, in this room full of brotherly love, I wonder where I've been for the last eleven months. No, that's not quite right. I know where I've been. I've been in denial after the shock of diagnosis, the rude indignities, the quick fixes that never worked. Why would I want to hang out with a bunch of old dudes, ignoring the fact that everybody dies in one way or another. We all know it but few are wise enough to believe it. Those who do rack up more precious moments than the entire population of fool's paradise, not to mention studies, studies showing those who do choose to be in a support group live years longer than the stiff upper lip recluse. And while I'm on the subject, I wonder where I'd be without the Internet, and the parade of dear supportive spirits met there in cyber-space, that mystical place where aid, care and concern are not determined by age, gender, race, physical appearance, economic situation or geological location. And this from a die-hard like me who not ten years ago held the computer in great disdain, convinced that poetry should be composed on the back of an envelope, with a blunt pencil while riding on a train. Thank God I'm past these prejudices, for without a support system I doubt if this recent malignant flare-up could have been withstood. How terrifying the thought of being at my writing desk disconnected, typing out memos to myself on my dead father's ancient Underwood.

—*In Support of Support Groups: A poem by a family member*

If at first you don't succeed,
try and try again.

—*Anonymous*

We cannot change anything unless we accept it.

—*Carl Jung*

Chapter 8: The Method

> The Lord is my shepherd
> I shall not want.
> He maketh me to lie down in green pasture.
> He leadth me besideth still waters.
> He restoreth my soul.
> He leadeth me in paths of righteousness
> For his name's sake.
> Yea, though I walk through the valley
> Of the Shadow of Death I fear no evil
> For Thou art with me,
> Thy rod and thy staff they comfort me.
> Thou preparest a table before me
> In the presence of mine enemies.
> Thou anointest my head with oil.
> My cup runneth over.
> Surely goodness and mercy shall
> Follow me all the days of my life
> And I will dwell in the house of the Lord
> Forever.
>
> —*Psalm 23*

The most encouraging observation I've made over all these years is that resilience is a strength most of us can develop with thought and practice.

—*Frederic Flach*

Everything in life that we really accept undergoes a change.

—*Katherine Mansfield*

A man was sleeping at night in his cabin when suddenly his room filled with light, and God appeared. The Lord told the man He had work for him to do and showed him a large rock in front of his cabin. The Lord explained that the man was to push against the rock with all his might. For years he toiled from sun up to sun down. Each night the man returned to his cabin sore and worn out, feeling his whole day had been spent in vain. Since the man was showing discouragement, Satan decided to enter the picture by placing thoughts into the weary mind: "You have been pushing against that rock for a long time, and it hasn't moved." The message was that the task was impossible and that he was a failure. These thoughts discouraged and disheartened the man. "Why kill myself over this?" he thought. "I'll just give the minimum effort." One day he decided to make it a matter of prayer and take his troubled thoughts to the Lord. "Lord," he said, "I have labored long and hard, putting all my strength to do that which you asked. Yet, after all this time, I have not even budged that rock. Why am I failing?" The Lord responded: "When I asked you to serve, I told you to push against the rock with all of your strength. Never did I mention I expected you to move it—just to push. And now you come to Me with your strength spent, thinking that you have failed. But, is that really so? Look at yourself. Your arms are strong and muscled, your back sinewy and brown, your legs have become massive and hard. Through opposition you have grown much and your abilities now surpass that which you used to have. Yet you haven't moved the rock." When everything seems to go wrong, just P. U. S. H. When people don't react the way you think they should, just P. U. S. H. When people just don't understand you, just P. U. S. H.   P=Pray U=Until S=Something H=Happens

—Anonymous

Don't fear failure so much that you refuse to try new things. The saddest summary of life contains three descriptions: 'could have,' 'would have,' and 'should have.'

—Louis E. Boone

Chapter 8: The Method

Honesty unbalanced by compassion is cruelty.
—*Tony Schwartz*

When life knocks you to your knees—
well, that's the best position in which to pray, isn't it?
—*Greta W. Crosby*

A just man falleth seven times and riseth up again.
—*Proverbs 24:16*

He only learns his freedom and existence
who daily conquers them anew.
—*Goethe*

Only the wounded healer heals.
—*T. S. Eliot*

What if you lived life as the miracle it is?
What would the day be like?
—*Herb Gravitz*

We either make ourselves miserable or we make ourselves strong.
The amount of work is the same.
—*Carlos Castaneda*

When one takes this journey of a lifetime and takes a disciplined approach to achieving it, there are some rather remarkable and predictable results for the family. As we have seen, however, they must begin within the person.

Each family member must get his or her wounds addressed. Strong family members create strong families. Just as a chain is as weak as its weakest link, the family is as strong as its strongest link. Strong members can overcome great obstacles. And overcoming great obstacles is exactly what is needed.

Let's look closer to find what many of the great thinkers have found that helps a family come back together after a major mishap. The interesting thing, of course, is that there is never coming back to anything—only moving forward toward something.

What we need to move forward to is arguably the most sacred of all institutions: the family. We can create healing and a triumphant family. We now have the knowledge. The rest is up to you. It is never too late to have a happy family. Perhaps more important, it is never too late to have a full life, as is described in my book *Mental Illness and the Family: Unlocking the Doors to Triumph*.

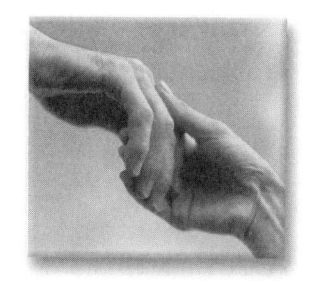

CHAPTER 9

Refamilying

There are few places indeed where any of us are not expendable. The family may be the one place on earth where none of us can be replaced. Paradoxically, it is also the place where most of us incur our greatest and deepest wounds, whether intentional or unintentional.

I will always remember one of the very early Adult Children of Alcoholics' conferences in which the distinguished psychiatrist, child advocate, and Holocaust survivor Dr. Bruno Bettelheim was the featured speaker. While I don't remember his exact words, he stated something like the following: To have a family is to have problems. He was proclaiming that problems are part of the very definition of family, a finding the reader should not be surprised by at this point in the book.

The relief I felt, however! The validation I experienced! All families have problems, the learned scholar proclaimed. This might sound strange, but for the first time I felt it was okay for me, too, to have family problems. Being a therapist is neither a guarantee of life's blessings nor of having first-rate personal coping skills to deal with life's major adversities. In fact, my favorite definition of a psychotherapist is someone who needs forty hours of therapy a week!

To accomplish this often not-easy task of triumphing over our problems and reconnecting with the family, each family member, to the best of his or her ability, must move through the stages of chaos, diagnosis, and core issues; then, move beyond the illness and "get himself or herself together."

We are reminded of this truism to take care of ourselves each and every time we fly on an airline. One of the very first things we hear is that "in the event of an unlikely drop in cabin pressure, an oxygen mask will drop down in front of you." Next, you are instructed to put it on first—even if you have an infant in your lap. The reason is quite simple, of course: unless you are in a resourceful place yourself, you will be of little help to anyone else. Put slightly differently, until your cup is full, it can't run over.

The focus of the book so far has been on you, the individual family member. Once you have understood the nature of your own wounds, have gone on your own personal odyssey, and acquired many of the tools you need, you are ready now to re-invest in the family in ways you never could. Recall that the third and final stage of the hero and heroine's journey is "the return" home. Like the great Greek warrior Odysseus, or Ulysses as he is sometimes called, you are now armed with all the shrewdness, skills, and knowledge of the journey that you will need to "re-family"(to family again, but from a very different place).

In this stage of family healing, there is a discovery or rediscovery of the miracle of "us." It is the affirmation of family power and a family way of coping with daily living and all the challenges it brings. It is the natural outcome of the previous stages. As family members get their lives together, they have the energy for family renewal. The possibility for a stronger and more vibrant family can now unfold. The needs of neither the primary nor the secondary sufferer no longer predominate; rather, the family becomes a place in which all members of the family are more able to grow and develop.

It is in this stage that the family is rebuilt, or developed. The past is released (and grieved) as everyone focuses on building a new and more positive future. New behaviors and new roles are becoming more stable. The illness, addiction, or other traumas now occupy less and less time and space in the lives of family members, and adversity is no longer the central organizing principle of the family.

It is not essential that the other family members "cooperate," or do things your way; what is important is that you are now able to be "in family" with yourself regardless of the external circumstances, which means loving in the presence of secure boundaries. The irony is that the more you can be with this possibility, the more likely it will be that the other members of the family actually cooperate.

So be sure to remember that, while not often a place of short-term comfort, families are around for the long haul of your life. You not only begin your life in a family, but, if you're lucky, you end your life in one as well. Public opinion polls show that having a good family life is one of the most important, if not the most important, goals in life for the vast majority of us. Perhaps something deep within us recognizes that the family is the foundation of civilization.

And by now, you may have begun to suspect that virtually regardless of your situation, it is never too late to have a happy family, a point that I make over and over again to all of the families I see. The more families I work with, the more convinced I become that virtually every family can be helped to some important degree. Love always leaves behind more than loss takes away.

> Home is the place where you belong,
> are accepted, understood, supported, and loved.
> Home is where people are interested in you.
>
> —*Pat Love*

> To be happy at home is the ultimate result of all ambition,
> the end to which every enterprise and labor tends.
>
> —*Samuel Johnson*

The first task of concerned people
is not to condemn or castigate or deplore;
it is to seek out the reason for disillusionment and alienation.
—Robert Kennedy

Your first and foremost job as a leader
is to take charge of your own energy
and then to help orchestrate the energy of those around you.
—Peter F. Drucker

The ability to control what we say when we're angry
is a prerequisite for a lasting relationship.
—Rabbi Joseph Telushkin

Home is the place where we can be ourselves and accept ourselves as both good and bad…where we can laugh and cry, where we can find some peace within all the chaos and confusion, where we are accepted and, indeed, cherished by others precisely because of our very mixed-up-edness. Home is that place where we belong, where we fit precisely because of our very unfittingness.
—Ernest Kurtz and Katherine Ketcham

In today's world great leaders are perhaps not best measured
by their success, but by how they deal with failure.
—Jon V. Peters

Chapter 9: Refamilying

> Success is 99 percent failure.
>
> —*Soichiro Honda*

> In great teams conflict becomes productive. The free flow of conflicting ideas and feelings is critical for creative thinking, for discovering new solutions no one individual would have come to on his own.
>
> —*Peter Senge*

> You don't know how good life can be,
> until you know how bad it can be.
>
> —*Ashleigh Brilliant*

> For what shall it profit a man if he should…
> gain the whole world and lose his soul?
>
> —New Testament

> Perhaps the greatest social service that can be rendered
> by anybody to the country and to mankind
> is to bring up a family.
>
> —*George Bernard Shaw*

> There is only one real deprivation…
> and that is not to be able to give
> one's gifts to those one loves most.
>
> —*Mary Sarton*

Family relationships provide our greatest heartaches.
But they also provide our greatest joys.
—David G. Myers

Everyone is a moon,
and has a dark side which he never shows to anybody.
—Mark Twain

Relationships that do not end peacefully do not end at all.
—Merrit Malloy

Eight out of ten people say we admire someone
who puts family before work.
—Recent Yankelovich poll

Love is forever; bitterness lasts only as long as we let it.
—William Blake

To be aware of a single shortcoming within oneself
is more useful than to be aware of a thousand in somebody else.
—Dalai Lama

The art of being wise is the art of knowing what to overlook.
—William James

Chapter 9: Refamilying

The test of a man or woman's breeding
is how they behave in a quarrel.

—*George Bernard Shaw*

Anybody can be angry. That is easy.
But to be angry with the right person, to the right degree,
at the right time, for the right purpose,
and in the right way, that is not easy.

—*Aristotle*

Strong relationships may be made in heaven,
but they need to be managed on earth.
That takes commitment, sharing, and tolerance—
and a host of refueling techniques.

—*Barrie Sanford Greiffe*

Be as a stone cast upon the water;
that the positive influence of your action
may extend far beyond the power of a mere pebble
in the hand of a man.

—*Ancient saying*

The measure of one's success in life is not the money raised.
It's the kind of family that is raised.

—*Joseph P. Kennedy*

Never give up on anybody.
—*Hubert H. Humphrey*

I never promised you a rose garden.
—*Hannah Green*

Tis easy enough to be pleasant,
When life flows along like a song;
But the man worthwhile is the one who will smile
When everything goes dead wrong.
—*Ella Wheeler Wilcox*

The bravest are surely those who have the clearest purpose…
and go out to meet it.
—*Thucydides*

Judge your success by what you had to give up
in order to get it.
—*Dalai Lama*

The holiest of all spots on earth
is where an ancient hatred has become a present love.
—*A Course in Miracles*

The family must be helped so that it can be resourceful enough to take on the illness. If the family is depleted, it won't have the strength to create an atmosphere counter to the atmosphere of the illness. Training the family frees up and releases the love, which is the fuel for the healing.

—*Herb Gravitz*

Everybody can be great...because anybody can serve.
You don't have to have a college degree to serve.
You don't have to make your subject and verb agree to serve.
You only need a heart full of grace. A soul generated by love.

—*Martin Luther King, Jr.*

It is more blessed to give than to receive.

—*Acts 20:35*

You have to do it by yourself, and you can't do it alone.

—*Martin Rutte*

Don't bug me! Hug me!

—*Bumper sticker*

Smile at each other, smile at your wife, smile at your husband, smile at your children, smile at each other—it doesn't matter who it is—and that will help you to grow up in greater love for each other.

—*Mother Teresa*

The glory of friendship is not so much in the outstretched hand or even in the kindly smile. It is in the spiritual inspiration that comes when you discover that someone else believes in you and is willing to trust you with his friendship.

—Ralph Waldo Emerson

Everybody likes a compliment.

—Abraham Lincoln

We have children to achieve biological immortality
or to meet family and societal expectations.
But we also have children to claim the opportunity
to shape another person's life.

—Rabbi Harold S. Kushner

We are who we love.

—Rabbi Harold S. Kushner

If a man could have half of his wishes, he would double his troubles.

—Benjamin Franklin

Our survival depends on the healing power of love,
intimacy and relationships....
I used to feel I was loved because I was special.
Now I feel special because I am loved and because I can love.

—Dean Ornish

We need people to tell us that we are special and irreplaceable, people who will tend to our needs and banish our fears and insecurities the way our mothers did when we were infants. But we also need to give love, to make a difference in someone's life.

—Rabbi Harold S. Kushner

And know here is my secret, a very simple secret; it is only with the heart that one can see rightly, what is essential is invisible to the eye.

—Antoine de Saint-Exupéry

Help your brother's boat across, and your own has reached the shore.

—Hindu proverb

You give before you get.

—Napoleon Hill

A saint would never be tempted to take the easy way, the more profitable way, enriching himself at the expense of others. A mensch [good person] would be sorely tempted but would resist the temptation. He would struggle with temptation but would prevail.

—Rabbi Harold S. Kushner

It is far better to establish a home than an opinion.

—Edmond Cabn

The quality of mercy its not strained;
It droppeth, as the gentle rain from heaven
Upon the place beneath; it is twice blessed;
It blesseth him that gives, and him that takes.
—William Shakespeare

We awaken in others the same attitude of mind
we hold toward them.
—Elbert Hubbard

Man becomes truly human
only at the time of decision.
—Paul Tillich

A great doctor works with an angel at her side.
—Folk saying

Who is a wise person?
One who learns from all people.
—Talmud

Listen and you will learn.
—Shlomo Ibn Gabirol

By emphasizing that which is good in people and in the world,
and by bringing the positive to the fore,
the evil is superseded by the good,
until it eventually disappears.

—*Rabbi Menachem Schneerson*

Much have I learned from my teachers,
more from my colleagues,
but most from my students.

—*Talmud*

You can give without loving,
but you can't love without giving.

—*Anonymous*

Our work brings people face to face with love.
To us what matters is an individual.
To get to love the person
we must come in close contact with him.

—*Mother Teresa*

There is a comfort in the strength of love;
t'will make a thing endurable,
which else would overset the brain or break the heart.

—*William Wordsworth*

We are all angels with only one wing.
We can only fly when we embrace each other.

—Old proverb

The highest form of wisdom is kindness.

—Talmud

Marriage is an edifice that must be rebuilt every day.

—André Maurois

Virtually every couple that had sex more often than they argued were happily married; no couple that had more fights than sex rated their marriage as happy.

—National Opinion Research Center's 1989 survey

He who loves brings God and the world together.

—Martin Buber

The family under the influence of illness,
addiction, or trauma can either be regarded as a POW
(prisoner of war) or in Basic Training—
Boot Camp in life and personal growth.

—Herb Gravitz

Chapter 9: Refamilying

> Love, that you may be loved.
> —*Moses Mendelssohn*

> We can do no great things;
> only small things with great love.
> —*Mother Teresa*

Someone once compared getting into an argument with a boorish neighbor to wrestling in the mud with a pig: You will both get filthy, but the pig will enjoy it. In any conflict, we have the option of walking away, not out of weakness or fear but out of strength, deciding that the price paid in gaining some satisfaction is more than we are willing to pay.
> —*Rabbi Harold S. Kushner*

> I keep my ideals, because in spite of everything,
> I still believe people are really good at heart.
> —*Anne Frank*

> Simply view yourself as a pioneer,
> in the long journey of increasing consciousness.
> —*Ken Keyes, Jr.*

> Our aspirations are our possibilities.
> —*Robert Browning*

> Love alone is capable of uniting living beings in such a way as to complete and fulfill them, for it alone takes them and joins them by what is deepest in themselves.
>
> —Pierre Teilhard de Chardin

> There is no good in arguing with the inevitable. The only argument available with an east wind is to put on your overcoat.
>
> —James Russell Lowell

> Our chief want in life is somebody who will make us do what we can.
>
> —Ralph Waldo Emerson

> Refusing to accept the alcoholic's denials and evasions, the family members can calmly and firmly tell him [the primary sufferer] that he has a disease, he needs help, and help is available. The alcoholic must know that the family is not bluffing, and the family should therefore be prepared to follow through on any threats made.
>
> —James Milam and Katherine Ketcham

> A slave is someone who does whatever her master wants. A servant is someone who does whatever the master needs, and it is she who decides what this might be.
>
> —M. Scott Peck

Chapter 9: Refamilying

> It's not how much you do,
> but how much love you put into the action.
>
> —*Mother Teresa*

> Independence?
> That's middle-class blasphemy.
> We are all dependent on one another—
> every soul of us on earth.
>
> —*George Bernard Shaw*

Peace must first be developed within an individual. And I believe that love, compassion, and altruism are the fundamental basis for peace. Once these qualities are developed within an individual, he or she is then able to create an atmosphere of peace and harmony. This atmosphere can be expanded and extended from the individual to his family, from the family to the community and eventually to the whole world.

—*Dalai Lama*

> For to let go of the ones who hurt us
> is to let go our identity as the one who was hurt,
> the one who was violated,
> the one who was broken.
>
> —*Rev. Wayne Muller*

> Judge not, that ye be not judged!
>
> —*Matthew 7:1*

Love is the only force capable
of transforming an enemy into a friend.
—Martin Luther King, Jr.

———

There can be no friendship
where there is no freedom.
Friendship loves a free air,
and will not be fenced up
in straight and narrow enclosures.
—William Penn

———

Love sought is good, but giv'n unsought is better.
—William Shakespeare

———

Our work is to keep our hearts open in hell.
—Stephen Levine

———

The ultimate measure of a man is not where he stands
in moments of comfort but where he stands
at times of challenge and controversy.
—Martin Luther King, Jr.

———

A professional is a man who can do his best
at a time when he doesn't particularly feel like it.
—Alistair Cooke

———

A teacher affects eternity;
he can never tell where his influence stops.

—*Henry Adams*

Use power to curb power.

—*Chinese proverb*

What you cannot enforce,
do not command.

—*Sophocles*

Leadership does not depend on being right.

—*Ivan Illich*

Leadership is the ability to get men to do
what they don't want to do and like it.

—*Harry Truman*

The absolute value of love makes life worthwhile,
and so makes Man's strange and difficult situation acceptable.
Love cannot save life from death;
but it can fulfill life's purpose.

—*Arnold J. Toynbee*

You can win more friends with your ears than your mouth.

—*Anonymous*

Love has nothing to do with what you are expecting to get—only what you are expecting to give—which is everything. What you will receive in return varies. But it really has no connection with what you give. You give because you love and cannot help giving. If you are very lucky, you may be loved back. That is delicious, but it does not necessarily happen.

—*Katherine Hepburn*

Who, being loved, is poor?

—*Oscar Wilde*

For unto whomsoever much is given,
of him shall be much required.

—*Luke 12:48*

It is a curious thought,
but it is only when you see people looking ridiculous,
that you realize just how much you love them.

—*Agatha Christie*

There is no remedy for love but to love more.

—*Henry David Thoreau*

Chapter 9: Refamilying

The good parent is he or she who keeps "showing up."
—*M. Scott Peck*

It takes two to make a quarrel, but only one to end it.
—*Spanish proverb*

A friend can tell you things you don't want to tell yourself.
—*Frances Ward Weller*

You can always tell a real friend:
when you've made a fool of yourself
he doesn't feel you've done a permanent job.
—*Lawrence J. Peter*

Shared joy is double joy, and shared sorrow is half-sorrow.
—*Swedish proverb*

Every man should have a fair-sized cemetery
in which to bury the faults of his friends.
—*Henry Brooks Adams*

Friends do not live in harmony merely,
as some say, but in melody.
—*Henry David Thoreau*

My best friend is the one who brings out the best in me.
—Henry Ford

People need loving the most when they deserve it the least.
—Mary Crowley

Making the decision to have a child—it's momentous.
It is to decide forever to have your heart go walking around
outside your body.
—Elizabeth Stone

I had only one friend, my dog.
My wife was mad at me,
and I told her a man ought to have at least two friends.
She agreed—and bought me another dog.
—Pepper Rodgers

Love possesses seven hundred wings,
and each one extends from the highest heaven
to the lowest earth.
—Jalaluddin Rumi

Love doesn't just sit there, like a stone,
it has to be made, like bread; remade all the time, made new.
—Ursula K. Le Guin

Chapter 9: Refamilying

The Eskimos had fifty-two names for snow because snow was important to them: there ought to be as many for love.

—Margaret Atwood

If you have built castles in the air, your work need not be lost; that is where they should be.
Now put the foundations under them.

—Henry David Thoreau

We need to restore the full meaning of that old word, duty. It is the other side of rights.

—Pearl S. Buck

Duty cannot exist without faith.

—Benjamin Disraeli

You will always find those who think they know what is your duty better than you know it.

—Ralph Waldo Emerson

In practice it is seldom very hard to do one's duty
when one knows what it is,
but it is sometimes exceedingly difficult to find this out.

—Samuel Butler

Somewhere along the line of development we discover what we really are, and then we make our real decision for which we are responsible. Make that decision primarily for yourself, because you can never really live anyone else's life, not even your own child's. The influence you exert is through your own life and what you become yourself.

—*Eleanor Roosevelt*

To know one's self is wisdom,
but to know one's neighbor is genius.

—*Anna Andrim*

The art of being wise is knowing what to overlook.

—*William James*

We often have to put up with most
from those on whom we most depend.

—*Baltasar Gracian*

The wise man forgets insults as the ungrateful forgets benefits.

—*Chinese proverb*

The salvation of mankind lies only in making everything
the concern of all.

—*Alexander Solzhenitsyn*

Chapter 9: Refamilying

Most of the good work of the world is done by people who weren't feeling all that well the day they did it.
—*Eleanor Roosevelt*

―◊―

A wise man hears one word and understands two.
—*Jewish proverb*

―◊―

I felt it shelter to speak to you.
—*Emily Dickinson*

―◊―

The pull of the future is as real as the pressure of the past.
—*Arthur Koestler*

―◊―

If there is a sin against life, it consists perhaps not so much in despairing of life as in hoping for another life and in eluding the implacable grandeur of this life.
—*Albert Camus*

―◊―

There is no direct connection between convenience and happiness.
—*Dr. Suzuki*

―◊―

When you truly possess all you have been and done, which may take some time, you are fierce with reality.
—*Florida Scott-Maxwell*

―◊―

> As for the Future, your task is not to foresee, but to enable it.
> All true creation is not a prejudgment of the Future…
> but the apprehending of a new aspect of the present.
>
> —William Bridges

This is the true joy in life, the being used for a purpose recognized by yourself as a mighty one; the being a force of nature instead of a feverish selfish little clod of ailments and grievances complaining that the world will not devote itself to making you happy. I am of the opinion that my life belongs to the whole community and as long as I live it is my privilege to do for it whatever I can. I want to be thoroughly used up when I die, for the harder I work the more I live, I rejoice in life for its own sake. Life is no "brief candle" to me. It is a sort of splendid torch which I have got hold of for the moment, and I want to make it burn as brightly as possible before handing it over to future generations.

—George Bernard Shaw

> If one person calls you a horse's ass,
> you can disregard it.
> If two people call you a horse's ass,
> you might want to think about it.
> If three people call you a horse's ass,
> get a saddle.
>
> —Yiddish proverb

> True happiness is not attained through self-gratification
> but through fidelity to a worthy purpose.
>
> —Helen Keller

Chapter 9: Refamilying

> Forget about like and dislike.
> They are of no consequence.
> Just do what must be done.
> This may not be happiness,
> but it is greatness.
>
> —George Bernard Shaw

> If you did nothing more when you have a family together than to make it possible for them to really look at each other, really touch each other, and listen to each other, you would have already swung the pendulum in the direction of a new start.
>
> —Virginia Satir

> I began to have an idea of my life, not as the slow shaping of achievement to fit my preconceived purposes, but as the gradual discovery and growth of a purpose which I did not know.
>
> —Johanna Field

> Even cowards can endure hardship;
> only the brave can endure suspense.
>
> —Mignon McLaughlin

> Living is a form of not being sure,
> not knowing what's next or how.
> The moment you know, you begin to die a little.
>
> —Agnes de Mille

Never have I enjoyed youth so thoroughly as I have in my old age.... Nothing is inherently and invincibly young except spirit. And spirit can enter a human being perhaps better in the quiet of old age and dwell there more undisturbed than in the turmoil of adventure.

—*George Santayana*

It's not how long it takes you to get there;
it is what you do once you arrive.

—*Variously attributed to Jesus and the Buddha*

To understand things we must have been once in them and then have come out of them; so that first there must be captivity and then deliverance, illusion, followed by disillusion, enthusiasm by disappointment. He who is still under the spell and he who has never felt the spell are equally incompetent

—*Amiel*

The best way to go fast is to go slow.

—*Herb Gravitz*

The Sufis say that real truth is always spoken with love, and that every word we speak must first pass through three gates: At the first gate we ask ourselves, "Are these words true?" If so we let them pass on. At the second gate we ask, "Are they necessary?" At the last gate we ask, "Are they kind?"

—*Sufi tale*

Never, never, never, never, never give up.

—*Winston Churchill*

Life is ten thousand joys and ten thousand sorrows.

—*The Buddha*

Every creature is a work of God.

—*Meister Eckhart*

The highest revelation is that God is in every person.

—*Ralph Waldo Emerson*

Treat a man as he is and he will remain as he is.
Treat a man as he can and should be
and he will become as he can and should be.

—*Goethe*

Cheerfulness, it would appear, is a matter which depends fully as much on the state of things within, as on the state of things without and around us.

—*Charlotte Brontë*

I am still determined to be cheerful and happy in whatever situation I may be, for I have also learned from experience that the greater part of our happiness or misery depends on our dispositions and not on our circumstances.

—Martha Washington

The best way to cheer yourself up
is to try to cheer somebody else up.

—Mark Twain

Be not deceived; God is not mocked:
for whatsoever a man soweth, that shall he also reap.

—Galatians 6:7

Nothing will content him who is not content with a little.

—Greek proverb

The secret of contentment is the realization that life is a gift, not a right.

—Anonymous

You can't have everything. Where would you put it?

—Steven Wright

Chapter 9: Refamilying

> To err is human, to forgive divine.
>
> —*Alexander Pope*

> We must develop and maintain the capacity to forgive. He who is devoid of the power to forgive is devoid of the power to love. There is some good in the worst of us and some evil in the best of us. When we discover this, we are less prone to hate our enemies.
>
> —*Martin Luther King, Jr.*

> The weak can never forgive.
> Forgiveness is the attribute of the strong.
>
> —*Mahatma Gandhi*

> Hard work is often an accumulation of the easy things you didn't do when you should have.
>
> —*Anonymous*

> Never refuse a good offer.
>
> —*Ancient proverb*

> The resilience literature points to
> the vital importance of mentoring:
> guiding and inspiring children in positive directions.
>
> —*Froma Walsh*

I like not only to be loved, but to be told I am loved.
—George Eliot

Loving life is living into an invented future
with one foot in reality.
—Mary Jo McGrath

Place a sick person in a healthy environment, and they will get better. Place a well person in a sick environment, and they will get worse.
—Anonymous

The cure for cynicism,
depression and narcissism is social action.
—Mary Pipher

Negotiation, of course, is at times impossible. The art of negotiation is a key to the family management of any major mental illness (in fact, any major chronic illness). One of the best books written on the art of negotiation comes from the Harvard Negotiation Project. It is called *Getting to Yes: Negotiating Agreement Without Giving In* by Roger Fisher and William Ury. Originally intended for application to business and diplomacy, this book is better than almost any psychology or family therapy text for learning how to negotiate effectively in families.

1. Separate the person from the problem. The idea is to get people's ego and pride disentangled from whatever the problem is so that the problem can be attacked without fear of attacking any person in the process.

2. Focus on interests, not positions. This is what separates negotiation from debating. A debating team defends—or attacks—a certain position, no matter what. It is its sole interest to be combative. Like an infantry, its position is its interest. Negotiation should never become debating (or trench warfare). In negotiation people have many interests, and it is the interests, not some debating position, that need to be satisfied. Indeed, one's position may sometimes go against one's interests and one does not want to be so identified with one's position that one cannot change it.

3. Generate a variety of possibilities before deciding what to do. This is particularly important in families under the influence, because it is the tendency of the person to bring premature closure to the discussion just to avoid the tension of the discussion itself. Don't feel everything has to be solved in one meeting. Get the problem out and let everybody take a few days to think about it, to come up with various options, and solutions.

4. Insist the result be based on some objective standard that ideally can be measured. This allows the members of the resolution to appeal the same standard other than their own will or opinion. Examples of objective standards might include: what do other families in this area do about this; what does the school recommend; what would the open market pay for this service or item; what is the relevant medical information regarding the safety of this activity.

—*The Harvard Negotiation Project*

Whenever you see a successful business,
someone once made a courageous decision.

—*Peter F. Drucker*

If we hold grudges, if we don't practice forgiveness, we end up stuck with the old grievances. It is only my attachment to the abuse that makes it my problem, once the actual abuse has stopped. In other words, my mind is perpetuating my own suffering.

—*Ram Dass*

Eleven characteristics that tend to differentiate families who cope well with stress from those who do not…include (1) clear acceptance of the stressor, (2) family-centered locus of the problem, (3) solution-oriented problem solving, (4) high tolerance, (5) clear and direct expressions of commitment and affections, (6) open and effective communication utilization, (7) high family cohesion, (8) flexible family roles, (9) efficient resource utilization, (10) absence of violence, and (11) infrequency of substance use.

—*Charles R. Figley*

Families who utilize dysfunctional coping methods…include (1) denial and misperception of the stressor, (2) individual-centered locus of the problem, (3) blame-oriented problem solving, (4) low tolerance, (5) indirect or missing expressions of commitment and affections, (6) closed and ineffective communication utilization, (7) low or poor family cohesion, (8) rigid family roles, (9) inefficient resource utilization, (10) utilization of violence, and (11) frequent use of substances.

—*Charles R. Figley*

Father, forgive them; for they know not what they do.

—*Jesus*

Chapter 9: Refamilying

> If we want to be heard
> we must speak in a language the listener can understand
> and on a level at which the listener is capable of operating.
>
> —*M. Scott Peck*

> There is no minimum at the start
> and there's no maximum at the end.
>
> —*Anonymous*

> The family is the major shock absorber between life and us.
>
> —*Herb Gravitz*

> We're a family again.
>
> —*Family members*

> My research found that the ratio of positive to negative interactions needed to exceed 10:1 for a marriage to be on a trajectory of increasing satisfaction.
>
> —*John Gottman*

> We cannot live only for ourselves.
> A thousand fibers connect us with our fellow men;
> and among those fibers, as sympathetic threads,
> our actions run as causes, and they come back to us as effects.
>
> —*Herman Melville*

It is in the shelter of each other that the people live.

—*Irish proverb*

From thee I receive
To thee I give
Together we share
That we both may live.

—*Family member*

We cannot solve the problems of today
with the same solutions that created them.

—*Albert Einstein*

We shall not cease from exploration
And the end of all our exploring
Will be to arrive where we started
And know the place for the first time.

—*T. S. Eliot*

Every time we work through some crisis, we get stronger. In a strange sort of way, we now see a crisis as a way of getting closer because we know what happens at the other end. I know it's weird, but it's also true. I guess—no I know—all the work is worth it.

—*Family member*

The psychological case for forgiveness is overwhelmingly persuasive. Not to forgive is to be imprisoned by the past, by old grievances that do not permit life to proceed with new business. Not to forgive is to yield oneself to another's control. If one does not forgive, then one is controlled by the other's initiatives, and is locked into a sequence of action, a response of outrage and revenge. The present is overwhelmed and devoured by the past. Those who do not forgive are those who are least capable of changing the circumstances of their lives. In this sense, forgiveness is a shrewd and practical strategy for a person or a nation to pursue, for forgiveness frees the forgiver.

—*Robin Casarjian*

History, despite its wrenching pain,
Cannot be unlived, and if faced with courage,
Need not be lived again.

—*Maya Angelou*

Where there is great love there are always miracles.

—*Willa Cather*

The sum total of our momentary feelings turns out to be a very flawed measure of how good or how bad we judge an episode—a movie, a vacation, a marriage, or an entire life—to be.

—*Martin Seligman*

Wisdom is knowing what to do, virtue is doing it.

—*David Starr Jordan*

Happiness is having a large, loving, caring,
close-knit family in another city.

—*George Burns*

Concern should drive us into action and not into a depression.

—*Karen Horney*

Joy shared is doubled and grief shared is halved.

—*Native American expression*

I have learned both to expect less from our daughter
and yet expect enough.

—*Family member*

The greatest roadblock to refamilying may be
the ability to leave a loved one to his or her own fate.

—*Herb Gravitz*

When you point your finger in blame,
there are three pointing back at you.

—*Anonymous*

All true benefits are mutual.

—*Elisabeth Kübler-Ross*

Chapter 9: Refamilying

> The only way to find out if you know
> is to call upon yourself to know.
>
> —Neale Donald Walsch

Love is patient, love is kind. It does not envy, it does not boast, it is not proud. It is not rude, it is not self-seeking, it is not easily angered, it keeps no record of wrongs. Love does not delight in evil but rejoices in the truth. It always protects, always trusts, always hopes, always perseveres. Love never fails.

> —1st Corinthians 13:4-8

> Be not angry that you cannot make others as you wish them to be since you cannot make yourself as you wish to be.
>
> —Thomas à Kempis

> I love you,
> Not only for what you are,
> But for what I am
> When I am with you.
>
> I love you,
> Not only for what
> You have made of yourself,
> But for what
> You are making of me.
>
> I love you
> For the part of me
> That you bring out.
>
> —Roy Croft

> Good people are good because
> they've come to wisdom through failure.
>
> —*William Saroyan*

> He who attempts to act and do things for others or for the world without deepening his own self-understanding, freedom, integrity and capacity to love, will not have anything to give to others. He will communicate to them nothing but the contagion of his own obsessions, his aggressiveness, his ego-centered ambitions, his delusions about ends and means, his doctrinaire prejudices and ideas.
>
> —*Thomas Merton*

> What would love do now?
>
> —*Neale Donald Walsch*

The ultimate triumph of the family is the experience of refamilying! Triumph and refamilying are both a cause and an effect of the healing of each family member and interact with each other synergistically.

Yet, there is little doubt that living under the influence of major illness, addiction, or other trauma may be one of the most harrowing tasks that any of us can endure in our life. More than one family member has quipped that their loved one would make even Gandhi loose his temper or Mother Teresa her patience. There can be a steady diet of unmet needs and serious disappointments. These are only a few of the many reasons why it is so essential to have other relationships that can support us when our loved ones cannot. And while we have also seen that these injuries may be the occasion for sacred wounding, which opens us to our true nature, the pain and anguishes that family members experience is no less present.

Perhaps most important, it is also because of the entire kaleidoscope of these occurrences, and not in spite of them, that we become open to the journey of a lifetime that all of the heroes before us undertook. Few say it more clearly than renowned mythologist Jean Houston, "As seed making begins with the wounding of the ovum by the sperm, so does soulmaking begin with the wounding of the psyche by the Larger Story."

Our role in our family is where so many of our "larger stories" take place. It is here that we first learn to deal with adversity and its strange and unlikely twin, triumph. We learn to deal with disappointment; we learn the importance and necessity of forbearance, perseverance, sacrifice, and tolerance; we learn that patience, compromise, and goodwill are the qualities that will make our lives consequential and meaningful.

In the environment of chronic illness, addiction, and other traumas, however, it is so easy to lose our bearings and, even worse, to lose ourselves. It may even be easier to feel victimized and faultless and to choose being right over being happy, a certain disaster in any intimate situation.

The New International King James Version of the Bible provides further instruction that is applicable to the wounding that this unholy alliance of illness, addiction, and other traumas brings and the refamilying it requires. For it would be inhuman not to feel righteous, angry, or the host of other equally strong and negative emotions that most family members experience. The New International Version in Ephesians 4:26, one of the Apostle Paul's letters to the first-century church at Ephesus, says, "Be angry, and do not sin."

There is such wisdom in these six words. For it is one thing to have an emotion and another to express it—especially in an unskillful and uninformed manner, which is characteristic of the early stages of family healing. It is crucial that family members walk the slippery slope between recognizing that all of their emotions and feelings are entirely normal and natural and at the same time not allow them to dictate their everyday behavior.

It is important to know that we may question whether refamilying is worth it. That is entirely normal and natural, too. Given that all families experience problems, given that families may be the only place where we are not replaceable, then I would like to suggest that it is almost always worth the effort to put the family together again after it has been torn apart by great adversity. When we are ready to leave this world and transition into the next, I don't think many of us will count our money, or any other possession for that matter. What we will do and whom we will think about most likely will relate to the people we have loved and the times we have spent with them.

Some may argue, however, that happiness or a happy family is an oversimplified, oxymoronic idea. When considering the idea of a full life, the following Sufi teaching provides yet another illuminating glimpse that offers all family members additional ways to place their circumstance in context: "The goal of man is Truth. Truth is more than happiness. The man who has Truth can have whatever mood he wishes, or none.... We have pretended that Truth is happiness and happiness Truth, and people have believed us. Therefore you, too, have until now imagined that happiness must be the same as Truth. But happiness makes you its prisoner, as does woe."

Therefore, I have found that family healing does not begin with correcting the communication and interaction patterns of the family so that the primary sufferer can recover, whether from illness, addiction, or other trauma. To the contrary, the healing capacity of the family is often reduced and the healing resources that are inherent within the family remain hidden when the family is approached in this manner. Rather, the healing of the family is an outgrowth and result of each individual family member's triumph.

Interaction is not always fun in any family. Producing a healthy family, let alone a happy family, more likely becomes a natural by-product and result of the healing of each family member. In the book, *Mental Illness and the Family: Unlocking the Doors to Triumph*, the distinction is made among a pleasant life, a good life, a meaningful life, and a full life. A full life is one that goes beyond a pleasant life, a good life, and even a meaningful life. It encompasses all three. A full life is a triumphant life, one in which all experiences are accepted by the individual, whether good or bad. The value of life goes beyond sensory pleasure, which is always temporary.

As I work with families, one of the most important questions that I suggest they ask themselves whenever they need to navigate a tricky and complicated situation is, "What would love do now?" This simple question brings forth the higher parts of us that can change instantly our perception of the situation and alter our attitude toward it. Neuroscience, the modern science of the brain, shows that questions such as these can literally alter the structure and function of the brain.

Life's constant play of opposites, victory and defeat, health and sickness, pleasure and pain, the best of times and the worst of times, are part and parcel of a life fully lived, a source of richness and depth rather than an obstacle or impediment when approached with compassion, understanding, and support.

In the final analysis, triumph, family healing, and a full life do not depend on the progress of any one family member, but the long overdue attention to all family sufferers. It is in this sense that a full life and a complete life are virtually always possible, regardless of circumstance. As such luminaries as Victor Frankl remind us, we have choices. Yet, our ability to deceive ourselves seems never-ending. I have discovered that the process of remembering this is less an end in and of itself than an ongoing challenge every day. For the helping professional, let alone the family, this is something we not only must teach but also live ourselves.

All family members are worthy and deserving in their own right of healing. Only when approached as the triumphant survivors that they can be, will family members become the tremendous resource that they are capable of being for each other. It is in this sense that refamilying can become a possibility worth striving for and that a full life is virtually always possible for individual family members.

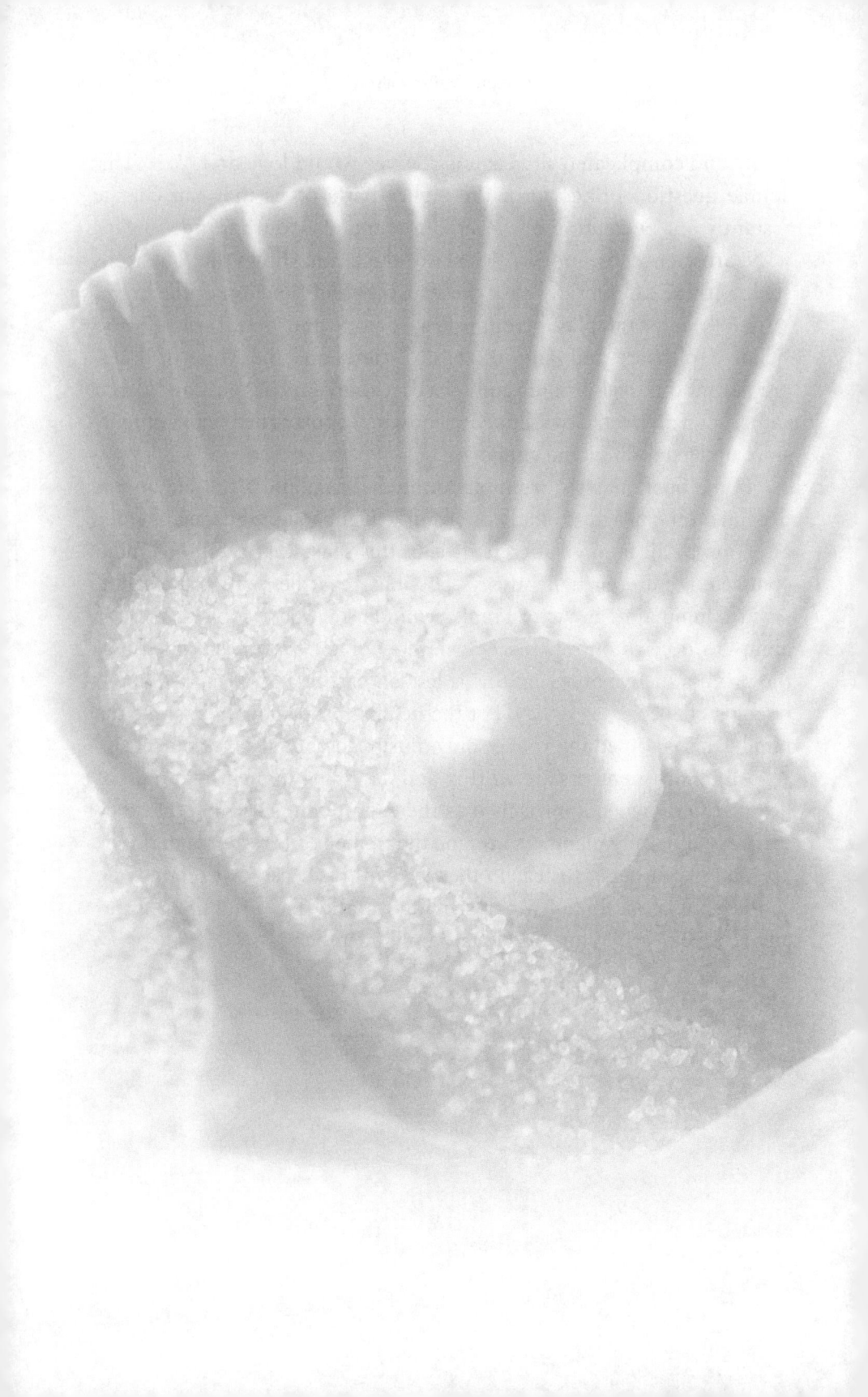

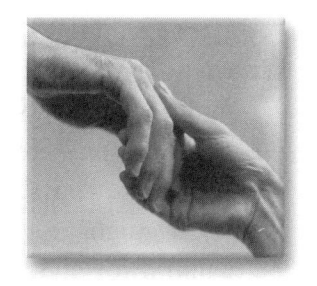

CHAPTER 10

The Outcome

The result of such a life's journey is what we take up now in our pursuit of words to heal every member of the family. However, the problems, solutions, and rewards of a life well-lived are not for the faint of heart. Such a life is truly the life for the modern hero and heroine. As a popular adage reminds us, "Life isn't for cowards and sissies."

The journey is an awesome one—just as are its fruits. It asks for no less of you than everything you have. It asks you to give up who you are now for the possibility of who you can become later. So some choose the devil they know rather than the devil they don't know.

As these words and sayings—these sound bytes for the soul—of mystics, poets, artists, scientists, researchers, clinicians, and family members have amply shown, diligence is its own reward. While the journey may seem daunting, it helps to know that it really is. That's why the sweetest fruit is out on the limbs.

But whenever I am beginning to learn a new skill that I know will take time, attention, and patience, I remember the words of one of my wisest teachers: "A few years from now," he used to say, "after you have learned this lesson, it will be the exact same few years from now during which you might not have even tried." Then, he'd add:

"And that would really be a tragedy, because what makes a tragedy a tragedy is that it often can be averted."

Another teacher, who taught me the fundamentals of working with people in altered states of consciousness, would softly say, "I wonder if you can thank yourself for giving yourself a new opportunity to learn what you might not have known before? And I wonder if you can be thankful for giving yourself the time it must take." And then, she would ever so gently add, "And I wonder if you can thank yourself for giving yourself the space to grow in." I must admit that it wasn't till months later that I really understood what she was asking me to do.

So I ask you: What better thing do you have to do with your time in the next few years? Have you really anything better to do with your time than devote yourself to the teachings of this "perennial philosophy," the truths that have withstood the tests of time and transcended cultures?

The next few years, which are about the amount of time it takes to incorporate these tenets, are going to pass, and pass quickly, no matter what you do. You might as well do something that you will be happy about later. Incidentally, I have often been asked how I arrived at the number, "a few years." It is because a few years are about the amount of time it takes to learn a foreign language well enough to dream in it.

So, if we do our work, if we take seriously the journey presented to us in these pages, then:

How will we emerge?
Will we be happy?
More happy than before?
Wise?
Healthy?
Wealthy?
Peaceful or mellow?
Or will we become defeated, demoralized, and dispirited?

As we have seen, it depends on us and on what we do, how we think, what we eat, what attitudes we cultivate, and with whom we do all of the above. And perhaps most importantly, it depends upon whether we listen to a "higher power" or a "lower power." Regardless, once again, the outcome is in our hands!

Chapter 10: The Outcome

> The highest reward from your working
> is not what you get for it but what you become by it.
>
> —*Sydney Harris*

> Almost all who become wiser and stronger after trauma
> do so because they develop a sense of purpose
> that transcends their immediate survival needs
> and allows them to focus on the future.
>
> —*Mary Pipher*

> Today is the first day of the rest of your life.
>
> —*Slogan from the children of alcoholics movement*

> One does not become enlightened by imaging figures of light, but making the darkness conscious.
>
> —*Carl Jung*

> As a psychiatrist, I feel it is important to mention at the outset two assumptions that underlie this book [*The Road Less Traveled*]. One is that I make no distinction between the mind and the spirit, and therefore no distinction between the process of achieving spiritual growth and achieving mental growth. They are one and the same. The other assumption is that this process is a complex, arduous and lifelong task.
>
> —*M. Scott Peck*

I may not be totally perfect, but parts of me are excellent.

—*Anonymous*

If you can grasp that the universe is made of nothing
continually turning into something,
then wearing plaids with prints comes easily.

—*Albert Einstein*

Security is mostly a superstition. It does not exist in nature, nor do the children of men as a whole experience it. Adding danger is no safer in the long run than outright exposure. Life is either a daring adventure or nothing.

—*Helen Keller*

The horizon leans forward offering you space
to place new steps of change.

—*Maya Angelou*

Effective help connects resources to problems
to achieve outcomes.

—*Herb Gravitz*

Momma always said
you gotta put the past behind you
before you can move on.

—*From the movie* Forrest Gump

Chapter 10: The Outcome

I went from thinking, "Good God, morning!"
to "Good morning, God!"

—*Family member*

—✠—

I have sometimes been wildly, despairingly, acutely miserable, racked with sorrow but through it all I still know quite certainly that just to be alive is a great thing.

—*Agatha Christie*

—✠—

The only reason you experience fear and disruption is
you are out of contact with the reality
of your own God consciousness.

—*Anamika*

—✠—

Everything is perfect,
but there is always room for improvement.

—*Suzuki Roshi*

—✠—

To think that life can still be good almost seems irreverent.

—*Family member*

—✠—

Since we are discovering that families who have received treatment do not develop new chemical dependencies, family treatment may be our best hope for preventing alcoholism and drug dependency in the next generation.

—*Sharon Wegscheider*

—✠—

It is never too late to give up your prejudices.
—Henry David Thoreau

Once we truly understand and accept it [life is difficult]—then life is no longer difficult. Because once it is accepted, the fact that life is difficult no longer matters.
—M. Scott Peck

You make me want to be a better man.
—Melvin Udall in the movie As Good As It Gets

I had to take a cab from Los Angeles to Santa Barbara, but only had $80 left for cab fare. I found a cab driver and asked him to take me as far as the $80 would go. He drove me as far as Ventura. When I got out, I gave him the $80. Then, I gave him a $10 tip. He looked surprised and said he thought that I only had $80. I said that was all I had for the fare, but I wanted to tip him, too. He told me to get back in the cab, and he drove me the rest of the way to Santa Barbara.
—Carl Grissanti

Each night, when I go to sleep, I die.
And the next morning when I wake up, I am reborn.
—Mahatma Gandhi

No great thing is created suddenly.
—Epictetus

Chapter 10: The Outcome

> The outcome depends more on the decisions one makes than the conditions one is under.
> —*Herb Gravitz*

> People are always blaming their circumstances for what they are. I don't believe in circumstances. The people who get on in this world are the people who get up and look for the circumstances they want, and, if they can't find them, make them.
> —*George Bernard Shaw*

> Who so loves
> Believes the impossible.
> —*Elizabeth Barrett Browning*

> Genuine love is volitional rather than emotional.
> —*M. Scott Peck*

> Courage is mastery of fear, not absence of fear.
> —*Mark Twain*

> The unexamined life is not worth living.
> —*Plato*

The curious paradox is that when I accept myself just as I am,
then I can change.
—*Carl Rogers*

No person is your friend who demands your silence,
or denies your right to grow.
—*Alice Walker*

The older I get,
the more I realize how many mistakes I make
and the less I care.
—*Family member*

Self-esteem comes from relative competence
rather than absolute control.
—*Herb Gravitz*

It is better to light a candle than to curse the darkness.
—*Chinese proverb*

It is easy enough to be friendly to one's friends.
But to befriend the one who regards himself as your enemy
is the quintessence of true religion.
The other is mere business.
—*Mahatma Gandhi*

Chapter 10: The Outcome

> God gives us our relatives;
> thank God we can choose our friends!
>
> —*Ethel Watts Mumford*

It is the consistent choice of the path with heart which makes the warrior different from the average man. He knows that path has heart when he is one with it, when he experiences a great peace and pleasure traversing its length.

> —*Carlos Castaneda*

> Take what you want said God and pay for it.
>
> —*Spanish proverb*

> I can trust my friends....
> These people force me to examine myself,
> encourage me to grow.
>
> —*Cher*

> The worship of God is not a rule of safety—
> it is an adventure of the spirit,
> a flight after the unattainable.
>
> —*Alfred North Whitehead*

> Maturity is the increasing ability to reconcile opposites.
>
> —*Carl Jung*

Sooner or later we all discover that the important moments in life are not the advertised ones, not the birthdays, the graduations, the weddings, not the great goals achieved. The real milestones are less prepossessing. They come to the door of memory unannounced, stray dogs that amble in, sniff around a bit, and simply never leave. Our lives are measured by these.

—Susan B. Anthony

The only way to have a friend is to be one.

—Ralph Waldo Emerson

Even if the doctor does not give you a year,
even if he hesitates about a month, make one brave push
and see what can be accomplished in a week.

—Robert Louis Stevenson

Freedom is what you do with what has been done to you.

—Jean-Paul Sartre

Friendship is not a fruit for enjoyment only,
but also an opportunity for service.

—Greek proverb

Freedom is feeling comfortable in harness.

—Robert Frost

Chapter 10: The Outcome

> I hate people who are intolerant.
> —*Laurence J. Peter*

> I desire to conduct the affairs of this administration that if at the end, when I come to lay down the reins of power, I have lost every other friend on earth, I shall at least have one friend left, and that friend shall be down inside of me.
> —*Abraham Lincoln*

> I set out to find a friend but couldn't find one;
> I set out to be a friend, and friends were everywhere.
> —*Anonymous*

> One or two thousand years ago when we spoke of a person's strength, we generally meant his physical strength: his capacity by virtue of pure musculature to beat other people up and hence rule over them or take their wives. Today when we talk of a person's strength we are usually doing so in purely psychological terms, specifically referring to his or her "strength of character."
> —*M. Scott Peck*

> It is not freedom from conditions
> but it is freedom to take a stand toward the conditions.
> —*Viktor Frankl*

> I have finally learned how little I really know—and it's okay.
> —*Family member*

There is a proper measure in all things,
certain limits beyond which and short of which
right is not to be found.

—Horace

Woe to him that claims obedience when it is not due;
woe to him that refuses when it is!

—Thomas Carlyle

If each one sweeps before his own door,
the whole street is clean.

—Jewish proverb

He that would be superior to external influences
must first become superior to his own passions.

—Samuel Johnson

There is a raging tiger inside every man
whom God put on this earth.
Every man worthy of the respect of his children
spends his life building inside himself
a cage to pen that tiger in.

—Murray Kempton

Angels can fly because they take themselves lightly.

—G. K. Chesterton

> A man's conquest of himself dwarfs the ascent of Everest.
>
> —*Eli J. Schaefer*

> The only person you can change is yourself.
>
> —*Alcoholics Anonymous slogan*

> There are nine requisites for contented living: health enough to make work a pleasure; wealth enough to support your needs; strength to battle with difficulties and overcome them; grace enough to confess your sins and forsake them; patience enough to toil until some good is accomplished; charity enough to see some good in your neighbor; love enough to move you to be useful and helpful to others; faith enough to make real the things of God; hope enough to remove all anxious fears concerning the future.
>
> —*Goethe*

> The man who views the world at fifty
> the same as he did at twenty
> has wasted thirty years of his life.
>
> —*Muhammad Ali*

> Wisdom is knowing what to do next;
> Skill is knowing how to do it, and Virtue is doing it.
>
> —*David Starr Jordan*

To have lived long does not necessarily imply the gathering of much wisdom and experience. A man who has pedalled twenty-five thousand miles on a stationary bicycle has not circled the globe. He has only garnered weariness.

—Paul Eldridge

Let us give thanks for this beautiful day. Let us give thanks for this life. Let us give thanks for the water without which life would not be possible. Let us give thanks for Grandmother Earth who protects and nourishes us.

—Daily prayer of the Lakota American Indian

You can't be brave if you've only had wonderful things happen to you.

—Mary Tyler Moore

In other words, the basic stuff of the universe, at its core, is looking like a kind of pure energy that is malleable to human intention and expectation in a way that defies our old mechanistic model of the universe—as though our expectation itself causes our energy to flow out into the world and affect other energy systems. Which, of course, is exactly what the third Insight would lead us to believe.

—The female protagonist in James Redfield's The Celestine Prophecy

What others think of you is none of your business.

—Ron Smith

Chapter 10: The Outcome

> Joy is not in things; it is in us.
> —*Richard Wagner*

> Sometimes even to live is an act of courage.
> —*Seneca*

> All wonders you seek are within yourself.
> —*Sir Thomas Browne*

Prigogine coined the term 'dissipative structures' to focus attention on the inherent contradiction of the two descriptors.... Dissipation describes a loss, a process by which energy gradually ebbs away. Yet Prigogine discovered that such dissipative activity could play a constructive role in the creation of new structures. Dissipation didn't lead to the demise of the system. It was part of the process by which the system let go of its present form so that it could reemerge in a form better suited to the demands of the present environment.

> —*Margaret Wheatley*

> Valor is a gift.
> Those having it never know for sure
> whether they have it till the test comes.
> And those having it in one test
> never know for sure if they will have it
> when the next test comes.
> —*Carl Sandberg*

Life is not so much a matter of holding good cards,
but sometimes of playing a poor hand well.

—Robert Louis Stevenson

The highest form of creativity is sculpting our life.

—Breck Costin

When you become the master of your mind,
nothing is good or bad, as such. All that is, is your destiny.

—Gurumayi Chidvilasananda

To be happy, one has to have something to live on, something to live for, and someone to live with. When one of them is missing, there is a challenge; when two are missing, it is drama and when all three are missing, you have tragedy.

—Sipreown Norwood

I have learned something really important throughout all of this tragedy. We don't have to become traumatized and assume the identity of a victim. You see, being a victim at first was out of my control. But avoiding the trap of a victimized lifestyle is now up to me. It is within my power the second time!

—Family member

Don't blame everything on the illness!

—Herb Gravitz

Peace is present right here and now, in ourselves and in everything we do and see. The question is whether or not we are in touch with it. We don't have to travel far away to enjoy the blue sky. We don't have to leave our city or even our neighborhood to enjoy the eyes of a beautiful child. Even the air we breathe can be a source of joy.

—*Thich Nhat Hanh*

A whole person is one who has both walked with God and wrestled with the devil.

—*Carl. G. Jung*

When we are no longer able to change a situation, we are challenged to change ourselves.

—*Viktor Frankl*

Without a sense of difference, without illness—events to counterpose health, health becomes nonexistent.... For without illness the fact of health is a contradiction in terms. For facts to be facts at all they first must be recognized. And, to be recognizable, they must stand out—here against a backdrop of periodic nonhealth, or illness.

—*Larry Dossey*

I altered my focus and immediately saw the energy fields around everything in my view.

—*The protagonist in James Redfield's* The Celestine Prophecy

"I can't believe that!" said Alice. "Can't you?" the queen said in a pitying tone. "Try again, draw a long breath, and shut your eyes." Alice laughed. "There is no use trying," she said. "One can't believe impossible things." "I dare say you haven't had much practice," said the queen. "When I was your age, I always did it for half an hour a day. Why, sometimes I've believed as much as six impossible things before breakfast."

—Lewis Carroll

Spiritually evolved people, by virtue of their discipline, mastery, and love, are people of extraordinary competence, and in their competence they are called on to serve the world, and in their love they answer the call.

—M. Scott Peck

Every day in every way, I'm getting better and better.

—Emile Coué

Pain, suffering, and grief will continue to be felt—but they will be attenuated, not magnified, by a new view of the world. We shall learn to participate in grief and pain from an utterly new perspective. It will be a perspective that modifies the meaning we impart to the experience, without eliminating the experience itself.... In such a process the fact of the experience remains; the event is not destroyed—it is the meaning that is imparted to it that is everything.

—Larry Dossey

Chapter 10: The Outcome

> Life is a song—sing it.
> Life is a game—play it.
> Life is a challenge—meet it.
> Life is a dream—realize it.
> Life is a sacrifice—offer it.
> Life is love—enjoy it.
>
> —*Sai Baba*

If anything, a realized soul is more in touch with the grief and sorrow that is part and parcel of the human condition, knowing that it too needs to be accepted and lived as all life needs to be lived. To reject the shadow side of life, to pass it by with averted eyes—refusing our share of common sorrow while expecting our share of common joy—would cause the unlived, rejected shadows to deepen in us as fear, including the fear of death.

—*Huston Smith*

> In a storm, it is the bamboo, the flexible tree,
> that can bend with the wind and survive.
> The rigid tree that resists the wind falls,
> victim of its own insistence to control.
>
> —*Joan Borysenko*

My religious faith…satisfies…the most fundamental human need of all. That is the need to know that somehow we matter, that our lives mean something, count as something more than just a momentary blip in the universe.

—*Rabbi Harold S. Kushner*

We've also pondered things that do enable happiness: fit and healthy bodies, realistic goals and expectations, positive self-esteem, feelings of control, optimism, outgoingness, supportive friendships that enable companionship and confiding, a socially intimate, sexually warm, equitable marriage, challenging work and active leisure, punctuated by adequate rest and retreat, a faith that entails communal support, purpose, acceptance, outward focus, and hope.

—David G. Myers

Nothing makes you happier than when you really reach out in mercy to someone who is badly hurt.

—Mother Teresa

If you want to become whole,
Let yourself be partial.
If you want to become straight
let yourself be crooked.
If you want to become full,
let yourself be empty.
If you want to be reborn,
let yourself die.
If you want to be given everything,
give everything up.

—I Ching

Resilience is not a once-and-for-all thing.
Our level of resilience will fluctuate over time.

—Frederic Flach

> If you want a definition of success, mine is short and sweet:
> Wake up and smell the coffee.
>
> —*Paul Pearsall*

Where you place your thoughts—which words you listen to, which words you allow to offer you direction and meaning—where you focus your attention, where you set your intention, all determine how successful you will be.

Dare to believe. The rest will follow.

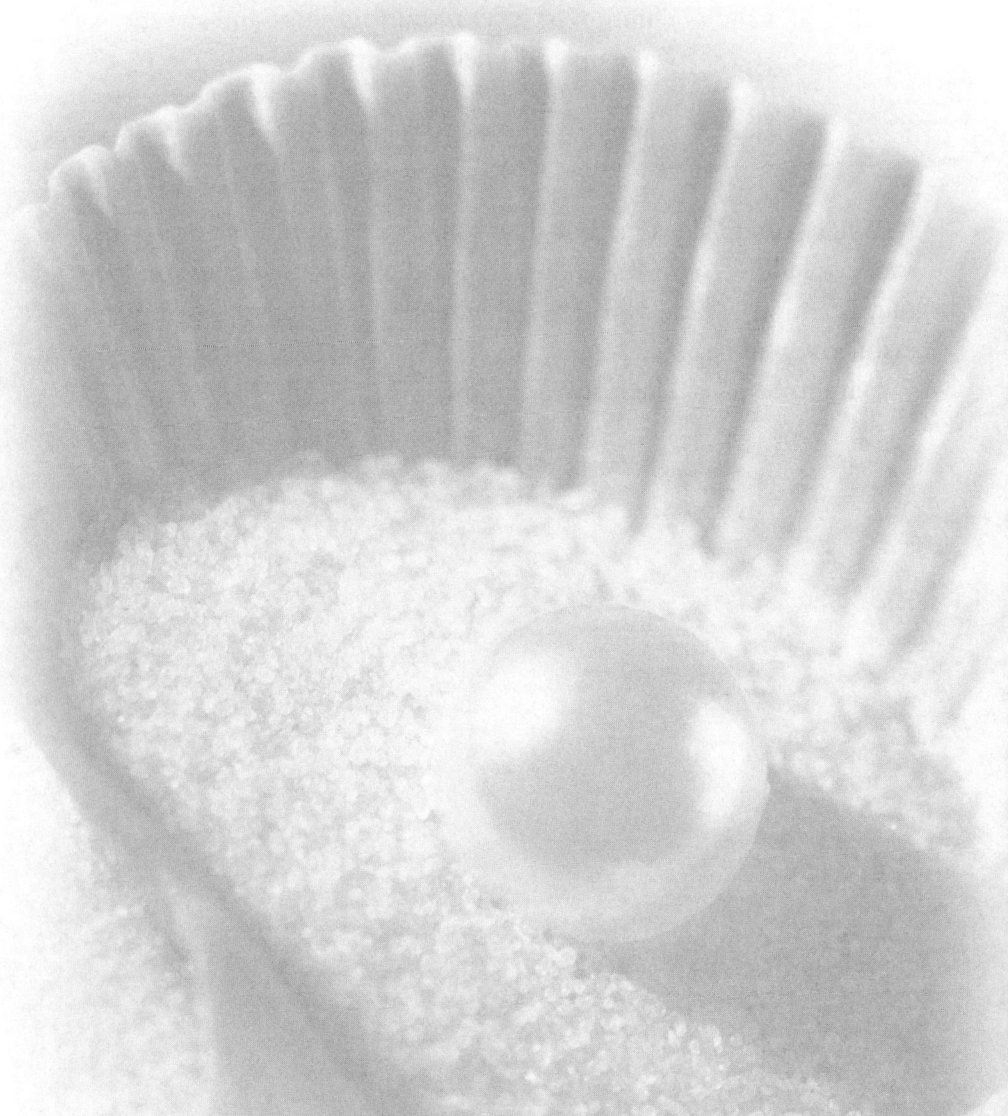

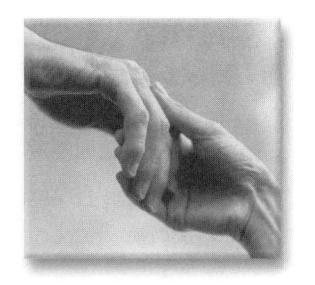

CHAPTER 11

Summary

Too few researchers and clinicians have considered the family as the source of resilience that it can be. Too many have neglected the family as a primary resource for hope and healing. The result has left many families overburdened, overwhelmed, and under-supported. Worse, the family can be left without a vision. And as the Bible reminds us, "Without a vision the people perish."

Hopefully, you now have a much wider lens through which to see the odyssey of every member of the family. Hopefully, you have a better appreciation not only of the problem, but, much more importantly, you have a new appreciation of the problem's potential and its solution. When the individual and family members work together in harmony, the family can return to its original place of safety for both the individual and society. It will take work and, as these collections of writings show, there is little doubt that we have the capacity to do it!

Highlights of the journey help us stay clear. They are our constant reminders of that upon which we most need to stay focused and centered. They keep us on the path. And whenever we wander—and whenever I wander, which admittedly is often—I take comfort in what one of my clients who is an airplane pilot told me. She said: "When an aircraft crosses the country, it is off course about 95 percent of the time, because the pilot can't control things like the wind, the weather, how much the people aboard weigh, how much their luggage weighs, and a host other important variables. The important thing," she emphasized, "is that the good pilot simply keeps the nose of the craft pointed in the direction of the flight plan."

We must remember to remember to keep the nose of our craft on the flight plan that each of us finds meaningful and fulfilling! It matters little that we are off course most of the time. It matters more how we respond, for all of life is—at its core—course correction!

The words of Vietnamese sage, peace activist, and poet Thich Nhat Hanh remind us of first things first. From this place of calm, we can proceed to understand and triumph over our adversities, regardless whether from illness, addiction, or other traumas. For, as we have seen, the results are remarkably similar—and so is the solution.

There is no knowledge that is not power.

—Ralph Waldo Emerson

There are two ways to live one's life—
as if nothing is a miracle, or as if everything is.

—Albert Einstein

No one can say of his house, "There is no trouble here."

—Asian proverb

Each self is a divine creation.

—*Sir John Eccles*

God made Truth with many doors
to welcome every believer who knocks on them.

—*Kahlil Gibran*

Above all we need to be taught more affection for the infirmities of life.... Both artist and lover know that perfection is not lovable. It is the clumsiness of a fault that makes a person lovable.

—*Joseph Campbell*

Happiness is not something someone gives you
but something you give yourself.

—*Spencer Johnson*

Every human being has the freedom to change at any instant....
A human being is a self-transcending being.

—*Viktor Frankl*

Mastery is less about forcing change upon the world around you
and more about redefining what your world means to you.

—*Gregg Braden*

Growing up means gaining the wisdom and skills to get what we want within the limitations imposed by reality—a reality which consists of diminished powers, restricted freedoms, and, with the people we love, imperfect connections.

—*Judith Viorst*

———

Getting everything we want is not the goal of healing nor does it necessarily spring from a sense of abundance. The mind, given free reign, will perpetually generate a lifetime of wants and desires, always wanting more and more and is never fully satisfied. Abundance arises when we feel that whatever we have is enough.

—*Dalai Lama*

———

The art of progress is to preserve order and change and to preserve change amid order.

—*Alfred North Whitehead*

———

You are here to enable the divine purpose of the universe to unfold. That is how important you are.

—*Eckhart Tolle*

———

I asked God how much time I had left and He answered, "Enough to make a difference."

—*Anonymous*

———

> Dance
> As though no one is watching you,
> Love
> As though you have never been hurt before,
> Sing
> As though no one can hear you,
> Live
> As though heaven is on earth.
>
> —*Alfred D' Souza*

There is a connection and fluidity to the events of life, not isolation and stasis, and these qualities make it impossible to superficially inspect a single happening and ascertain its goodness or badness.... Life then ceases to be a disjunctive sequence of the good and the bad, but becomes a unitary phenomenon.

—*Larry Dossey*

> The love in our hearts,
> when embraced, when extended,
> has the miraculous power to change the course of events.
>
> —*Marianne Williamson*

> Breathing in, I calm body and mind.
> Breathing out, I smile.
> Dwelling in the present moment
> I know this is the only moment.
>
> —*Thich Nhat Hanh*

Love is all you need.
—*The Beatles*

Get a life.
—*Anonymous*

You never know what opportunities
are just around the corner.
—*Family member*

The best things in life are free.
—*Anonymous*

Compassion can be our world's richest energy source.
—*Matthew Fox*

Love, it turns out,
may be one of the most powerful
physical forces in the universe.
—*Diane Goldner*

Live as if you will die tomorrow,
Learn as if you will live forever.
—*Mahatma Gandhi*

> Great stories always begin in a wasteland
> and small stories always end there.
>
> —*Joseph Campbell*

> Life deals the hand, but we have to play it.
>
> —*Family member*

> Humans are like tea bags; you have to put them in hot water
> before you know how strong they are.
>
> —*Sophie Gravitz*

> Nothing is too wonderful to be true.
>
> —*Michael Faraday*

> It is important to remember that you are not responsible for becoming ill, and you are not responsible for your recovery. What you are responsible for once you are ill is to do your best to get better.
>
> —*Lawrence LeShan*

> Like a modern-day Jonah,
> the person (family) under the influence of illness, addiction,
> and trauma is swallowed by a whale of an experience.
>
> —*Herb Gravitz*

What is frequently ignored by the pop psychology movement is that, in the "body-mind-spirit" composite that is used to refer to man, spirit is radically beyond health. It includes all qualities, because it is subject to no dualisms. It is, thus, healthy and unhealthy, and is paradoxically, all other sets of contrast we can devise…. [thus] the highest spiritual state is patently not the same as perfect physical health. The domains are different—because one is ultimate and excludes nothing…. That is why we have seen and continue to see mystics die young, and why great spiritual masters contract tuberculosis, intestinal parasites, hemorrhoids, and athlete's foot like the rest of us—and why they also laugh about it…. And still the temptation must be resisted over and over, that of turning "higher health" which exists at the spiritual level into "perfect health" at the material, bodily level…. Perfect bodily health is not given out with spiritual enlightenment like so many Green Stamps, a bonus for being good or for "making it." Higher health cares not a whit for (although it includes) numerical values of the cholesterol level, the amplitude and frequency of one's brainwaves, or the duration spent in twitchless relaxation.

—*Larry Dossey*

When you are standing very close to a large object, all you can see is the object. Only by stepping back from it can you also see the rest of its setting around it. When we are stunned by some tragedy, we can only see and feel the tragedy. Only with time and distance can we see the tragedy in the context of a whole life and a whole world.

—*Rabbi Harold S. Kushner*

Grant me the courage to serve others;
for in service there is true life.

—*César Chávez*

The full circle of spiritual truth will be completed
only when we realize that,
but for a destiny not fully understood,
we might actually have been born in the other person's faith.

—*Marcus Bach*

The struggle for health is a struggle against fragmentation and disunity. Health in its fullest form involves the capacity to accept the whole—in the certain knowledge that all the experiences of life cohere in a locked interdependence, connected to each other for their very meaning.

—*Larry Dossey*

A moment's insight is sometimes worth a life's experience.

—*Oliver Wendell Holmes*

God gives us gifts and they are often wrapped in problems.

—*Philip B. Gravitz*

Life is a long lesson in humility.

—*J. M. Barrie*

No man is an island, entire of itself;
every man is a piece of the Continent,
a part of the main.

—*John Donne*

If you want to know what God is all about,
try giving Him the benefit of the doubt.

—*Anonymous*

Hope is the feeling you have
that the feeling you have isn't permanent.

—*Jean Kerr*

We are not human beings trying to be spiritual.
We are spiritual beings trying to be human.

—*Jacquelyn Small*

Every man is a damn fool for at least five minutes every day.
Wisdom consists in not exceeding the limit.

—*Elbert Hubbard*

The road to wisdom? Well, it's plain
And simple to express;
Err
And err
And err again
But less
And less
And less.

—*Piet Hein*

We are surrounded with insurmountable opportunities.

—*Pogo Possum*

You must create your own world.
I am responsible for my world.

—*Louise Nevelson*

Almost every wise saying has an opposite one,
no less wise, to balance it.

—*George Santayana*

It's taken me all my life to understand
that it is not necessary to understand everything.

—*Rene Coty*

What is most important to keep in mind is that research has consistently demonstrated that the prognosis for individuals with serious mental illnesses improves when family members are provided with the information and support they need as caregivers.

—*Herb Gravitz*

Happiness must be cultivated. It is like character.
It is not a thing to be safely let alone for a moment,
or it will run to weeds.

—*Elizabeth Stuart Phelps*

I know of no more encouraging fact
than the unquestionable ability of man
to elevate his life by conscious desire.
—Henry David Thoreau

All suffering prepares the soul for vision.
—Martin Buber

In the midst of winter,
I finally learned that there was in me an invincible summer.
—Albert Camus

The mouse that has but one hole is easily captured.
—Norma and Philip Barretta

The mind is its own place, and in itself
Can make a heav'n of hell, a hell of heav'n.
—John Milton

Sex is the most fun you can have without laughing.
—Woody Allen

I have found my hero and he is me.
—George Sheehan

Chapter 11: Summary

> Carpe diem. (Seize the day.)
> —*Horace*

> Keep your eye on the donut, not the hole.
> —*Norma and Philip Barretta*

> Just do it!
> —*Family member*

> No one really knows enough to be a pessimist.
> —*Norman Cousins*

> While I breathe, I hope.
> —*Ancient proverb*

> Do unto others, as you would have them do unto you.
> —*Anonymous*

> Do unto others as you would have them do unto you, but only if you were in their unique and very different shoes.
> —*M. Scott Peck*

Amazing grace! How sweet the sound,
That saved a wretch like me;
I once was lost, but now I'm found;
Was blind, but now I see.

—*John Newton*

If you think you'll lose, you're lost,
For out in the world we find
Success begins with a fellow's will;
It's all in the state of mind.
Life's battles don't always go
To the stronger or faster man;
But soon or later the man who wins
Is the man who thinks he can.

—*Walter D. Wintle*

God grant me the serenity to accept the things I cannot change, the
courage to change the things I can,
and the wisdom to know the difference.

—*Serenity Prayer*

Faith is to believe what you do not yet see;
the reward for this faith is to see what you believe.

—*Saint Augustine*

Believe those who are seeking the truth; doubt those who find it.

—*André Gide*

When in doubt, gallop.
—*Motto of French Foreign Legion*

We keep encountering the same issues again and again, but from a wiser place.
—*Herb Gravitz*

Neurosis is always a substitute for legitimate suffering.
—*Carl Jung*

Great is the gate and narrow is the way which leadeth to life, and few there be who find it.
—*Jesus*

Truth is one; the sages speak of it by many names.
—*The Vedas*

Life gives us moments, and for those moments we give our lives.
—*Anonymous*

Here's a test to find whether your mission on earth is finished: If you're alive, it isn't.
—*Richard Bach*

Commit random gestures of kindness,
perform senseless acts of beauty.
—Anonymous

Be content with your lot.
One cannot be first in everything.
—Chinese fortune cookie

Build a future; don't try to save a past.
—Herb Gravitz

Life always gets harder towards the summit.
—Friedrich Nietzsche

We are here to do,
And through doing to learn;
and through learning to know;
and through knowing to experience wonder;
and through wonder to attain wisdom;
and through wisdom to find simplicity;
and through simplicity to give attention;
and through attention
to see what needs to be done.
—Rabbi Ben Hei Hei

Chapter 11: Summary

It's never too late to have a happy family.

—*Sophie Gravitz*

It ain't over 'til it's over.

—*Yogi Berra*

There's this little wave, a he-wave who's bobbing up and down in the ocean off the shore, having a great time. All of a sudden, he realizes he's going to crash into the shore. In this big wide ocean, he's now moving toward the shore, and he'll be annihilated. "My God, what's going to happen to me?" he says, a sour and despairing look on his face. Along comes a female wave, bobbing up and down, having a great time. And the female wave says to the male wave, "Why are you so depressed?" The male says, "You don't understand. You're going to crash into that shore, and you'll be nothing." She says, "You don't understand. You're not a wave; you're part of the ocean."

—*Morrie Schwartz*

To affect the quality of the day, that is the highest of action.

—*Henry David Thoreau*

One of the greatest ironies is that stressful lives often provoke positive emotions while easier lives can induce laziness and apathy. Who is happier, a mountain climber or a person who sits around and watches television all weekend?

—*Mary Pipher*

The fate of American families must be viewed as a national problem, and, as such, it is the responsibility of federal and state governments to intervene in revitalizing troubled families. Just as government neglect has undermined the infrastructure of the family, it will take substantial federal support to reverse long-term processes that have been contrary to the health of families and, thus, to the well-being of us…the fates of societies and families are intertwined.

—David A. Karp

To express our deepest Self is the greatest purpose of life.

—Herb Gravitz

Health is like wealth.
Although its utter absence can breed misery,
having it is no guarantee of happiness.

—David G. Myers

There are two dogs inside me.
One of the dogs is mean and evil. The other dog is good.
The mean dog fights the good dog all the time.

—Native American expression

We might not have a choice about whether we have been victimized, but we do have a choice about whether we become victims.

—John Goulet

You've failed many times, although you may not remember. You fell down the first time you tried to walk. You almost drowned the first time you tried to swim, didn't you? Did you hit the ball the first time you swung a bat? Heavy hitters, the ones who hit the most home runs, also strike out a lot. R. H. Macy failed seven times before his store in New York caught on. English novelist John Creasey got 753 rejections slips before he published 564 books. Babe Ruth struck out 1330 times, but he also hit 714 home runs. Don't worry about failure. Worry about the chances you miss when you don't even try.

—Message in the Wall Street Journal
by United Technologies Corporation

—∞—

Learning is finding out
What you already know.
Doing is demonstrating that you know it.
Teaching is reminding others that they know it just as you.

—Richard Bach

—∞—

The sun is always shining somewhere.

—Family member

—∞—

Ever tried. Ever failed.
No matter.
Try again. Fall again. Fall better.

—Samuel Beckett

—∞—

So what kind of people are we? Are we naturally good and pure until external circumstances compromise our goodness. Or are we naturally weak and deceitful, needing conscious or outside authority to keep us in line? My answer is that we are both.

—Rabbi Harold S. Kushner

Resilient people tell themselves a story
that gives their lives meaning and purpose.

—Mary Pipher

It is pretty hard to tell what does bring happiness.
Poverty and wealth have both failed.

—Ken Hubbard

…which may serve to show us that it is the mind, and not the sum, that makes any person rich…. No one can be poor that has enough, nor rich, that covets more than he has.

—Seneca

Finding the occasional straw of truth awash in a great ocean of confusion and bamboozle requires intelligence, vigilance, dedication and courage. But if we don't practice these tough habits of thought, we cannot hope to solve the truly serious problems that face us—and we risk becoming a nation of suckers, up for grabs by the next charlatan who comes along.

—Carl Sagan

Chapter 11: Summary

> Everything can be taken from a man but one thing;
> the last of the human freedoms—
> to choose one's attitude in any given set of circumstances,
> to choose one's own way.
>
> —*Viktor Frankl*

> Live a good, honorable life.
> Then when you get older and think back,
> you can be able to enjoy it a second time.
>
> —*Dalai Lama*

> To repeat, if we seek greater serenity we can strive to restrain our unrealistic expectations, to go out of our way to experience reminders of our blessings, to make our goals short-term and sensible, to choose comparisons that will breed gratitude rather than envy.
>
> —*David G. Myers*

> And now let us welcome the New Year
> Full of things that have never been.
>
> —*Rainer Maria Rilke*

> Four Phrases to Live By:
> Thank you.
> I love you.
> How are you?
> What do you need?
>
> —*Rabbi Jack Riemer*

Symptoms of Inner Peace:
A tendency to think and act spontaneously rather than on fears based on past experiences. An unmistakable ability to enjoy each moment. A loss of interest in judging other people. A loss of interest in interpreting the actions of others. A loss of interest in conflict. A loss of the ability to worry. (This is a very serious symptom). Frequent, overwhelming episodes of appreciation. Contented feelings of connectedness with others and nature. Frequent attacks of smiling. An increasing tendency to let things happen rather than make them happen. An increased susceptibility to the love extended by others as well as the uncontrollable urge to extend it.

—*Cherie Carter-Scott*

When I was young, I set out to change the world. When I grew a little older, I perceived that this was too ambitious, so I set out to change my state. This, too, I realized as I grew older, was too ambitious, so I set out to change my town. When I realized that I could not even do this, I tried to change my family. Now as an old man, I know that I should have started by changing myself. If I had started with myself, maybe then I would have succeeded in changing my family, the town, or even the state—and who knows, maybe even the world!

—*Old Hasidic tale*

If we saw ourselves as God sees us, we would smile a lot.

—*Anonymous*

Whoever saves a single life is as if one saves the entire world.

—*Talmud*

To remove those living in this life from the state of misery and lead them to the state of felicity. At the beginning it is horrible and fetid; for it is Hell; and in the end it is prosperous, desirable, and gracious, for it is Paradise.

—*Dante Alighieri*

The serious problems in life…are never fully solved. If ever they should appear to be so it is a sure sign that something has been lost. The meaning and purpose of a problem seems to be not in its solution but in our working at it incessantly.

—*Carl Jung*

We have taken a long journey together. It is a journey that in its essence is quite simple. Would that it be as easy.

We have addressed many problems and have covered many issues through the words of some of the greatest minds of all times. Now, the rest is up to you.

I wish you well on your life's journey. Be mindful, however, that quote after quote can become tedious unless you remember to pause often. Go slowly. Be deliberate. You may even want to return to some of these sayings again and again. They can be like a very rich dessert. They are to be savored. Rest often. Gather the fruits of your labor. And be sure to smell the flowers along the way.

Dare to be inspired and breathe in the spirit and wisdom of the ages. The result can be healing and triumph beyond your imagination.

Bon voyage and let the good times roll.

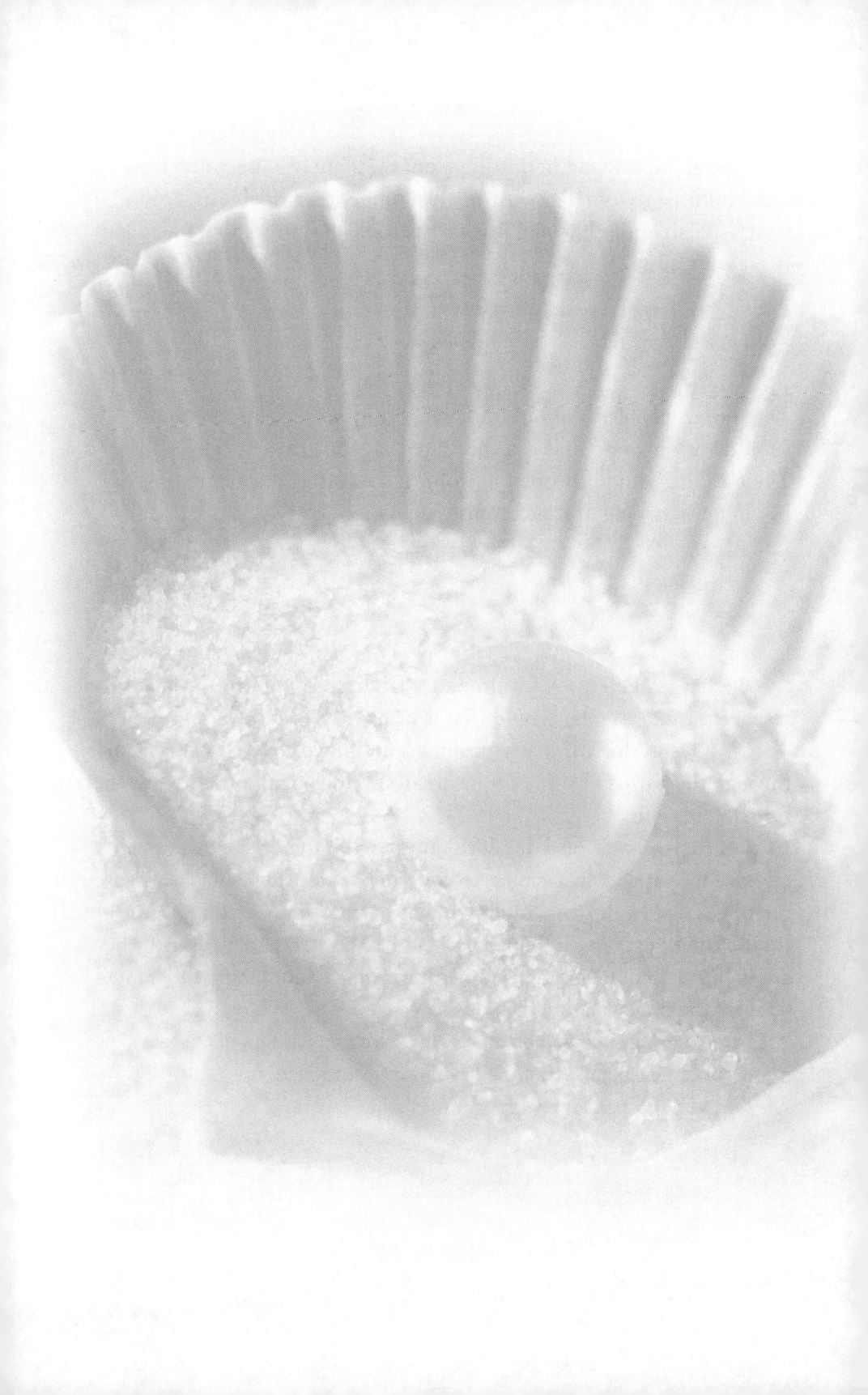

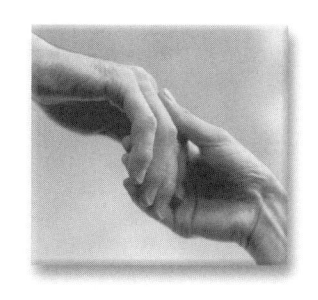

Postscript

—⚬—

Endings are never easy, even when we have surrendered to the fact that they are also new beginnings. That withstanding, it is time to close.

In thinking about which words to conclude our journey together, those that kept returning to me were uttered by spiritual guides who span the past, the present, and the future: the first are from Lao Tzu, who lived more than two thousand years ago; the second are from St. Francis of Assisi, the founder of the Franciscans, who lived in the thirteenth century; the third are from Dorothea Dix, the noted nineteenth-century advocate for the mentally ill; the fourth are from Neale Donald Walsch, who is a twenty-first century spiritual guide; the fifth from Gregg Braden, known as a weaver of the ancient texts with modern science; and the last is from John Schaar, the distinguished futurist.

I leave you, my reader, with their thoughts.

—⚬—

Begin difficult things
While they are easy,

Do great things
When they are small,

The difficult things of the world
Must once have been easy;

The great things
Must once have been small . . . .

A thousand mile journey
Begins with
A single step.

—*Lao Tzu*

Lord make me an instrument of thy peace.
Where there is hatred, let me sow love;
Where there is injury, pardon;
Where there is doubt, faith;
Where there is despair, hope;
Where there is darkness, light;
Where there is sadness, joy.

O divine Master, grant that I may not so much seek
To be consoled as to console,
To be understood as to understand,
To be loved as to love;
For it is in giving that we receive;
It is in pardoning that we are pardoned;
It is in dying to self that we are born to eternal life.

—*Saint Francis of Assisi*

> They say, "Nothing can be done here!"
> I reply, "I know no such word in the vocabulary I adopt!"
>
> —Dorothea Dix

So when a particular thing happens to you, don't ask yourself why it is happening. Choose why it is happening. Decide why it is happening. If you can't choose or decide with intention, then make it all up. You are anyway. You are making up all the reasons for doing things, or for why things are happening the way they are. Yet most often you are doing this unconsciously. Now make up your mind (and your life) consciously!

—Neale Donald Walsch

Quantum science suggests the existence of many possible futures for each moment of our lives. Each future lies in a state of rest until it is awakened by choices made in the present.

—Gregg Braden

The future is not a result of choices among alternative paths offered by the present, but a place that is created—created first in mind and will, created next in activity. The future is not some place we are going to, but one we are creating. The paths to it are not found but made, and this activity of making them changes both the maker and the destination.

—John Schaar

What is important about the principles espoused by all of these messengers of wisdom is the invitation to make use, consciously and with intention, of your inherent ability to participate in the creation of your own life story. This story consists of beliefs that carry our thoughts. Anything created is created first as thought. The more energy we put into the thought, the more likely it is that you will attract that reality to you. Thought is energy and it can actually be measured. Look to who you are being as you express the energy of thought in meaningful action.

As you weave the strands together from all of the wisdom teachers and wisdom keepers of all times in a way that is personally meaningful, you participate in a journey that continues throughout life.

Best wishes on this special journey.

Remember to remember that the true winners in life know that the journey is never a sprint. It is always a marathon.

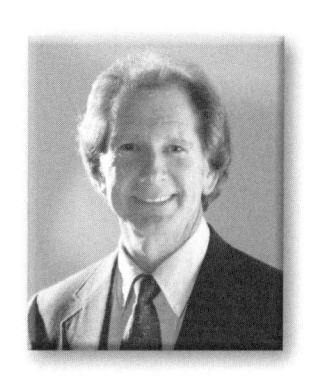

About the Author

Herbert L. Gravitz, Ph.D., received his Master's Degree and Doctor of Philosophy in psychology from the University of Tennessee in 1969. A licensed psychologist, his private practice in clinical psychology is located in Santa Barbara, California. He specializes in the diagnosis and treatment of the effects of illness, addiction, and other trauma on the individual, the family, and society. He is known for his innovative work in systemic traumatology, specifically the impact on the individual and the whole family of alcoholism, post-traumatic stress disorder (PTSD), obsessive-compulsive disorder (OCD), bipolar disorder, major depression, and schizophrenia.

Dr. Gravitz has authored or co-authored books and articles on trauma, healing, and recovery, and he has led workshops and seminars throughout the United States on the traumatic impact of alcoholism and major mental illness on the family. He is the co-author of *Recovery: A Guide for Adult Children of Alcoholics,* a modern classic in the field of children of alcoholics, and he is co-author of *Genesis: Spirituality in Recovery from Childhood Traumas.* He authored *Obsessive Compulsive Disorder: New Help for the Family,* which has received overwhelming endorsement from professionals and organizations, as well as individuals and their families.

His most recent book, *Mental Illness and the Family: Unlocking the Doors to Triumph*, provides a groundbreaking approach for families to triumph over the impact of mental illness and other major life adversities.

Dr. Gravitz is completing two new books. The first, *Trauma and Adversity: Triumph's Crucible*, shares in depth his pioneering synthesis of the fields of trauma, addiction, loss and grief, altered states of consciousness, physical healing, mythology, personal excellence, the new sciences, the energy therapies, and spirituality—all of which lead to a powerful healing transformation. The second book, *Bittersweet: Cancer as a Sacred Wound*, utilizes all the principles in his last book plus new insights from working with families under the influence of cancer, an overwhelming illness that affects virtually every family. He and wife Leslie, also a writer and educator for 30 years, are working on this book together to bring hope and help to every member of the family under this devastating illness.

The website for Dr. Gravitz is www.HealTheFamily.com, and his e-mail address is mail@HealTheFamily.com.

Dr. Gravitz' message of hope and optimism regarding the impact of illness, addiction, and trauma on both the individual and the family makes him a frequent guest on radio and television. In addition to his busy private practice in Santa Barbara, he is a Founding Member of the Board of Directors of the National Association of Children of Alcoholics (NACoA) and served on its Advisory Board. He is also a Founding Member of the Board of Directors of The Memory to Action Project, a not-for-profit organization whose mission is to commemorate genocide, encourage tolerance, and promote commitment to social action. He holds Diplomates in Psychotherapy, Traumatic Stress, and Forensic Psychology. In addition, he is Board Certified in Illness Trauma by the American Academy of Experts in Traumatic Stress.

Dr. Gravitz' first professional experience with people suffering from mental illness occurred following his first year of graduate school, when he worked as a psychiatric aide at Chestnut Lodge, an internationally known residential treatment center in Rockville, Maryland.

He did his clinical internship at Larue D. Carter Memorial Hospital in Indianapolis, Indiana, in 1968, where he worked with the seriously mentally ill in an in-patient setting. From 1972 to 1980, while first Assistant Director and later Program Director of the University of California at Santa Barbara Counseling Center, he worked extensively with students who experienced serious mental illness. When he entered private practice in 1980, he counseled the seriously mentally ill and their families in his role as Psychological Consultant to Sanctuary House. Sanctuary House was started as an alternative residential treatment program for the seriously mentally ill, and it became a nationally respected treatment facility that continues to serve the needs of the mentally ill and their families. While at Sanctuary House, he formed the first group psychotherapy program for its residents and frequently consulted with family members. In 1983, he served as a consultant to the Santa Barbara Psychiatric Emergency Team where he provided staff development.

It was not until the early 1990s that Dr. Gravitz became aware of how many clients in his outpatient private practice also were the family members of those who suffered from serious mental illnesses, such as schizophrenia, bipolar disorder, major depression, obsessive-compulsive disorder, or some other severe illness. By the middle of the 1990s, he began to describe the plight of the family that was living under the influence of mental illness.

Because illness, addiction, and trauma often occur together in the same family, Dr. Gravitz has learned to address all three in unique ways that go beyond traditional family approaches. In this process, he has discovered ways to speak simultaneously to the sufferer and to the sufferer's loved ones. Dr. Gravitz routinely began to treat the family as a whole in the late 1990s, regardless of how many family members were actually present in a session. He continues to forge new frontiers in his intensive and creative consultations. In this regard, he is known for his innovative intergenerational treatment protocols and his pioneering work in "untimed" consultation sessions, in which the family works on an issue until everyone present agrees it is time to stop.

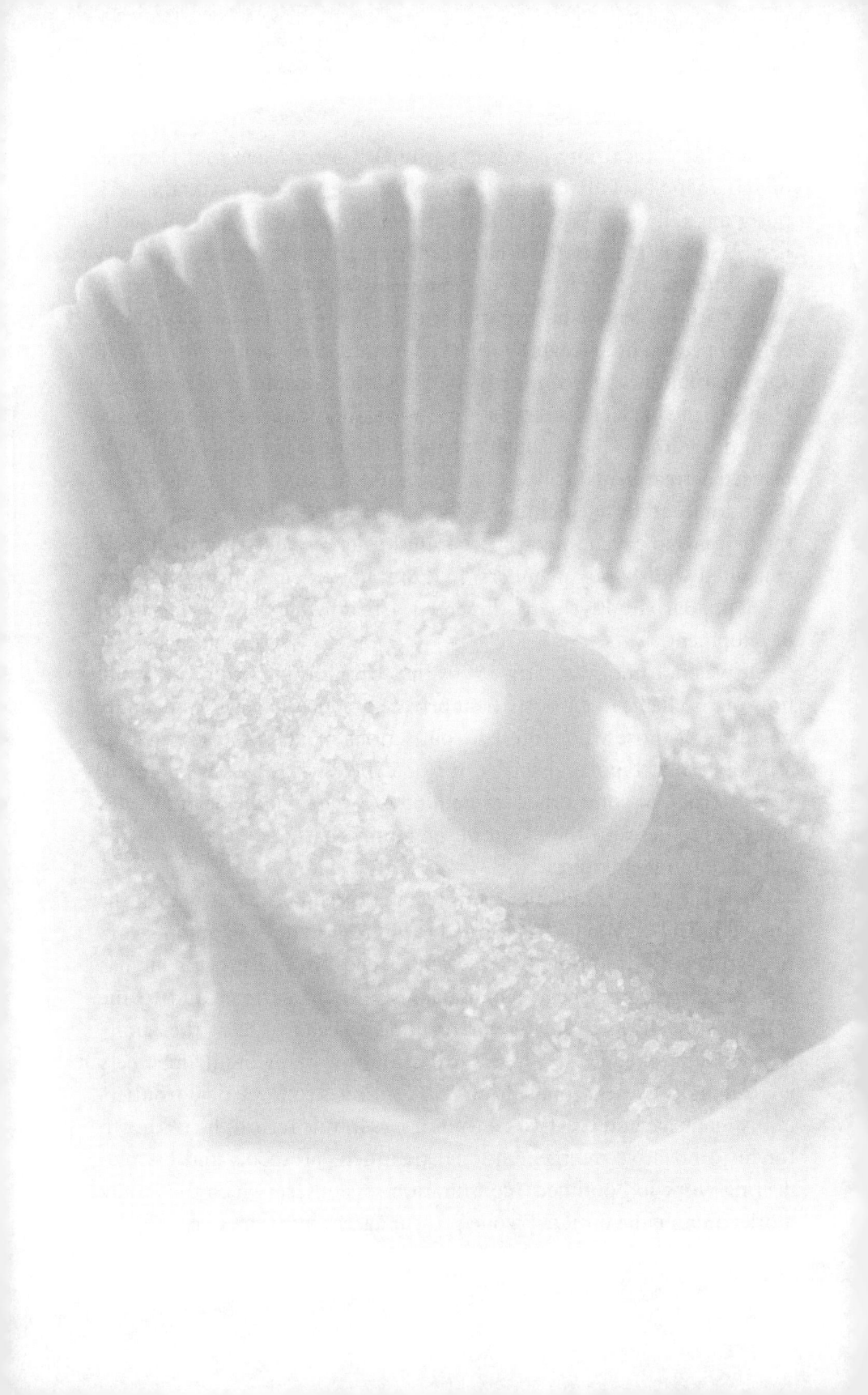

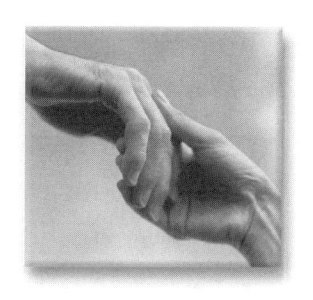

Partial List of Contributors

Many of the contributors of these inspiring quotes are well known to most readers and need little or no introduction. Some names, however, may be unfamiliar, and thus it might be useful to have these very brief sketches about some of the contributors.

Joseph Addison—noted English writer

Alcoholics Anonymous—12-Step Program for the alcoholic and the very first of a number of 12-Step programs

Al-Anon—family organizational wing of Alcoholics Anonymous for the family and friends of those under the influence of alcohol

Louisa May Alcott—author of classics such as *Little Women*

Muhammad Ali—former heavyweight champion boxer once known as Cassius Clay

Robert and Jane Alter, Ph.D.s—specialists and authors in trauma psychology

Anamika—contemporary clairvoyant, mystic, awakened teacher

Susan B. Anthony—famous historical figure in the women's rights movement

Guillaume Apollinaire—French poet

Aristotle—ancient Greek philosopher

Mary Kay Ash—multi-millionaire and founder of Mary Kay cosmetics

Marcus Aurelius—Roman statesman and philosopher

Richard Bach—author of such modern classics as *Robert Livingston Seagull*

Francis Bacon—English philosopher known for the saying, "Knowledge is power"

Mary Catherine Bateson, Ph.D.—noted author and workshop leader in the human potential movement

Gregory Bateson, M.D.—noted author, psychiatrist, and anthropologist

The Beatles—perhaps the greatest rock-and-roll band of all times

Henry Ward Beecher—noted African-American author

Claude Bernard, M.D.—physician noted for the concept of "homeostasis"

Claudia Black, Ph.D.—one of the founders of the children of alcoholics movement

Robert Bly—noted American poet and leader in the men's movement

Gregg Braden—author, lecturer, and guide to sacred sites throughout the world regarding ancient wisdom, planetary change, and the role of relationships within the context of these changes

General Omar Bradley—World War II U.S. general

John Bradshaw—noted author, lecturer, and subject of PBS series on the family, inner child, and addiction

Nathaniel Branden, Ph.D.—noted author and lecturer on self-esteem and romantic love

William Bridges, Ph.D.—consultant and lecturer on the topic of transitions and executive development

Ashleigh Brilliant—contemporary American humorist

Erin Brockovich—environmental activist about whom a movie was made

Rita Mae Brown—author noted for the saying, "insanity is doing the same thing over and over and expecting different results"

Robert Browning—poet

Pearl S. Buck—American author of such classics as *The Pearl*

George Burns—renowned American comedian

Joseph Campbell, Ph.D.—noted mythologist, especially for his writings on the Hero's Journey

Richard Carlton—Former CEO, 3M Corporation

Dale Carnegie—one of the original self-help gurus

Thomas Carlyle—famous British poet and philosopher

Johnny Carson—TV comedian and former talk-show host

Cherie Carter-Scott—entrepreneur, lecturer, seminar leader, and chairperson of the board of Motivation Management Service Inc.

Carlos Castaneda—author of the *Tales of Don Juan*

César Chávez—activist and champion of civil rights

Cher—singer, actress, comedian

G. K. Chesterton—British writer

Agatha Christie—famous mystery writer

Confucius—Chinese philosopher and founder of Confucianism

Emile Coué—famous French psychiatrist known for the statement, "Every day in every way, I am getting better and better"

Course in Miracles, A—modern spiritual classic

Norman Cousins—wrote the classic, *Anatomy of An Illness*, a layperson's use of humor and self-responsibility to cure what doctors said was an incurable disease

Harvey Cushing, M.D.—noted early physician

Dalai Lama—the great spiritual leader of Tibet

Ram Dass—formerly Richard Alpert of Harvard University who has become a leading spokesperson for spirituality and advocate of "fierce grace"

Diagnostic and Statistical Manual of Mental Disorders, **Fourth Edition**—commonly called *DSM-IV*, the "bible" of psychiatric diagnoses

Kenneth Doka, Ph.D.—well-known writer on death, dying, and grieving

John Donne—noted sixteenth-century English theologian and poet

Larry Dossey, M.D.—new-age physician known for Level III medicine and the power of prayer

Peter F. Drucker—pre-eminent management scholar

Karlfried Graf Durckheim—famous sociologist noted for concept of "anomie"

Thomas Edison—famed discover and inventor of such things as the electric light bulb

Albert Einstein, Ph.D.—great twentieth-century physicist and discoverer of theory of relativity

Dwight David Eisenhower—noted general and former president of the United States

T. S. Eliot—famous American poet who wrote the classic "Wastelands"

Emmanuel—mystic and spiritual medium

Epictetus—great Roman philosopher who wrote what is probably the first self-help book

Epicurus—ancient philosopher

William J. Everett—noted theologian

Marilyn Ferguson, Ph.D.—noted futurist and author

Marshal Ferdinand Foch—famed military leader

Charles R. Figley, Ph.D.—noted psychologist and trauma specialist

St. Francis of Assisi—famed Franciscan monk who is the saint of humility, charity, and love

Viktor Frankl, M.D.—noted psychiatrist and survivor of concentration camps who started Logotherapy

Robert Frost—great American poet

John Galsworthy—English novelist

Kahlil Gibran—Sufi poet and author of *The Prophet*

André Gide—French novelist

Goethe—famous German poet and author of *Faust* and other classics

Diane Goldner—contemporary author of science and spirituality

John Goulet, M.A.—marriage and family therapist in Ventura, California

Philip Benjamin Gravitz—my father

Sophie Korim Gravitz—my mother

Carl Grissanti—family friend

Hamlet—one of William Shakespeare's most famous plays

Stephen Hawking, Ph.D.—one of the world's leading contemporary physicists

Ernest Hemingway—noted fiction writer

Harville Hendrix, Ph.D.—noted author, lecturer, and psychologist on love and marriage and the family

Katernine Hepburn—former movie great and Academy Award-winning actress

Judith Herman, Ph.D.—noted feminist and traumatologist

Rabbi Hillel—famous Jewish rabbi of antiquity

Soichiro Honda—founder of Honda Motor Company

Horace—great Roman poet and philosopher

Jean Houston, Ph.D.—well-known lecturer and author on sacred psychology and the further possibilities of human functioning

Lee Iacocco—famous American businessman

I Ching—famous Chinese classic of practical wisdom

Ivan Illich—Russian author on illness, particularly iatrogenic illness

William James, Ph.D.—the father of American psychology

Samuel Johnson—English dramatist known to have been a sufferer of a variety of mental illnesses

Richard Kammann—the late New Zealand researcher in happiness

David A. Karp, Ph.D.—noted sociologist and expert on family impact of mental illness

Charlotte Davis Kasl, Ph.D.—psychologist, healer, and author whose emphasis is on women, addiction, and trauma

John Keats—famed seventeenth-century English poet

Helen Keller—the deaf and blind woman who has come to be an inspiration for millions

Joseph Kennedy—famous father of John F. Kennedy

Ben Kenobi—the Jedi master in the classic movie *Star Wars*

Charles Kettering—American inventor

Soren Kierkegaard—noted existential Swedish philosopher

Rudyard Kipling—great British poet and author

Henry Kissinger, Ph.D.—former Secretary of State in Nixon administration

Elisabeth Kübler-Ross, M.D.—the noted psychiatrist whose groundbreaking 1969 book, *On Death and Dying*, changed the world's view of the dying process, lifting the taboo from the study of thanatology, and spawning the founding of the American hospice movement

Bessel A. van der Kolk, M.D.—noted Harvard psychiatrist and expert on traumatic stress

The Koran—the Islamic Bible

Lao Tzu—ancient Chinese philosopher and founder of Taoism

D. H. Lawrence—noted British author of fiction

Sam Levenson—American humorist

Martin Luther King, Jr.—famous civil rights leader and Nobel Peace Prize winner

Henry Wadsworth Longfellow—one of America's best-loved poets

Pat Love, Ph.D.—family and marriage therapist and relationship expert

Antonio Machado—Spanish poet and school teacher

Machiavelli—author of the classic, *The Prince*

Moses Maimonides—perhaps the greatest Jewish philosopher and theologian, who wrote during the medieval period

Gideon Markman, Ph.D.—Assistant Professor of Entrepreneurship, Lally School of Management and Technology, Rennselaer Polytechnic Institute

Rollo May, M.D.—well-known psychiatrist and author of numerous classics in the area of psychotherapy

Golda Meir—former Prime Minister of Israel

H. L. Mencken—political satirist

Henry Miller—noted American author

John Milton— next to Shakespeare, regarded as greatest English poet

Wilson Mizner—American humorist

Montage—French poet and philosopher

Mary Tyler Moore—contemporary American comedian and actress

Rev. Wayne Muller—best-selling author and minister on spiritual aspects of healing

Gerald D. Myers, Ph.D.—noted researcher on the science of happiness

Reinhold Niebuhr—credited as author of the "Serenity Prayer"

Friedrich Nietzsche—noted German philosopher

Anaïs Nin—one of the leading women writers of the twentieth century

Dean Ornish, M.D.—widely respected modern physician and researcher on the effects of lifestyle on health

Rosa Parks—famous for her pioneering role in integrating the South

Blaise Pascal—contemporary of Descartes, who was a brilliant philosopher and mathematician

Cesare Pavese—Italian writer

Norman Vincent Peale—well-known inspirational author of self help classics, *How to Win Friends and Influence People* and *The Power of Positive Thinking*

M. Scott Peck, M.D.—author and psychiatrist whose best-selling book, *The Road Less Travelled*, is a modern-day spiritual classic

Jon V. Peters—president, The Institute for Management Studies

Mary Pipher, Ph.D.—psychologist and best-selling author on the family

Plato—ancient Greek philosopher

Pogo Possum—cartoon character noted for wisdom and saying the obvious

Carol Primeau, Ph.D.—psychologist in Santa Barbara, California

Sumner Redstone—Chairman of the Board, Viacom, Inc.

Cheri Register—expert, sufferer, and author on the effect of chronic illness on the family and loved ones

Eddie Rickenbacker—famous World War I pilot

Sally Ride—noted woman astronaut

Rainer Maria Rilke—famous German poet

John D. Rockefeller, Jr.—American entrepreneur and financier

Carl Rogers, Ph.D.—one of the most influential psychologists of all time and founder of client-centered therapy

John S. Rolland, M.D.—noted author and expert on the impact of chronic illness on the family

Eleanor Roosevelt—noted for her humor, insight, and wisdom, she was the wife of Franklin D. Roosevelt

Franklin D. Roosevelt—former president of the United States

Galen Rowell—international photographer and mountaineer

Miguel Ruiz—author and philosopher of Toltec wisdom

Jalaluddin Rumi—well-known Sufi poet and philosopher

Bertrand Russell—British philosopher, logician, essayist, and critic

Babe Ruth—famous Hall of Fame baseball player and home run hitter

Oliver Sacks, M.D.—contemporary author of modern classics on neurology

Carl Sagan, M.D.—philosopher, scientist, and author

Antoine de Saint-Exupéry—French novelist

George Santayana—philosopher noted for the statement, "Those who cannot remember the past are condemned to repeat it"

Jean-Paul Sartre—poet and existential philosopher

David Satcher, M.D.—Surgeon General of the United States

Albert Schweitzer, M.D.—humanitarian, theologian, and physician

Secondary sufferers of illness, addiction, and trauma—the neglected affected or family and friends of those suffering from a major chronic illness

Victoria Secunda—lecturer and author on the impact of mental illness on the family

Martin P. Seligman, Ph.D.—noted psychologist for his work on learned helplessness, optimism, and positive psychology

Seneca—the first-century Stoic philosopher

Shakespeare—one of the greatest writers and dramatists of all time

George Bernard Shaw—famous British author and playwright

Susan Skog—contemporary journalist and author who has interviewed and profiled many of today's prominent spiritual authors and teachers

Gerald L. Sittser, Ph.D.—associate professor of religion whose story of the tragic loss of his whole family is an inspiration to all

Song of Solomon—well-known verse in the Bible

Alexander Solzhenitsyn—Nobel Prize-winning Russian author

Susan Sontag, M.D.—noted psychiatrist

Sophocles—ancient Greek philosopher and dramatist

Benjamin Spock, M.D.—beloved physician who gave advice to countless parents for decades

Elaine St. James—popular, contemporary writer on the topic of living simply

Adlai E. Stevenson—former statesman and presidential candidate

Tom Stoppard—American dramatist

Dr. Suzuki—renowned Zen master

Albert Szent-Gyorgyi, M.D., Ph.D.—twice Nobel Prize laureate

Rabindranath Tagore—Nobel Prize laureate and one of India's greatest poets

Talmud—collection of Jewish wisdom

Joseph Telushkin—contemporary rabbi, spiritual leader, scholar, and author

Mother Teresa—twentieth-century saint known for her loving care of the poor and injured

Margaret Thatcher—former prime minister of Great Britain

Thich Nhat Hanh—Nobel Prize-winning Buddhist poet and philosopher

Robert Thomsen—author of the biography of *Bill W.*, who is the co-founder of Alcoholics Anonymous

Eckhart Tolle—contemporary mystic, writer, and philosopher, who wrote the classic book, *The Power of Now*

Lily Tomlin—noted American comedian

Arnold J. Toynbee, Ph.D.—renowned British historian

Mark Twain—noted American humorist and essayist

Evelyn Underhill—well-known nineteenth-century writer and mystic

The Vedas —ancient Hindu texts

Judith Viorst, Ph.D. —best-selling author and psychologist

Froma Walsh, Ph.D. —noted psychologist and expert on family resilience

Neale Donald Walsch —best-selling author of the *Conversations with God* trilogy

Booker T. Washington —the foremost educator and leader of African-Americans at the turn of the twentieth century

Thomas J. Watson, Sr. —founder of IBM

Sharon Wegscheider —noted pioneer in the field of the impact of alcoholism on the family

Margaret Wheatley, Ph.D. —well-known author and organizational consultant

Alfred North Whitehead, Ph.D. —famous physicist

Oscar Wilde —flamboyant British dramatist and playwright

Marianne Williamson —international author and teacher in the fields of spirituality and new thought who teaches the basic principles of *A Course in Miracles*

John P. Wilson, Ph.D. —contemporary researcher and author in the traumatic stress field

Marion Woodman, M.D. —noted author and lecturer on addiction and spirituality

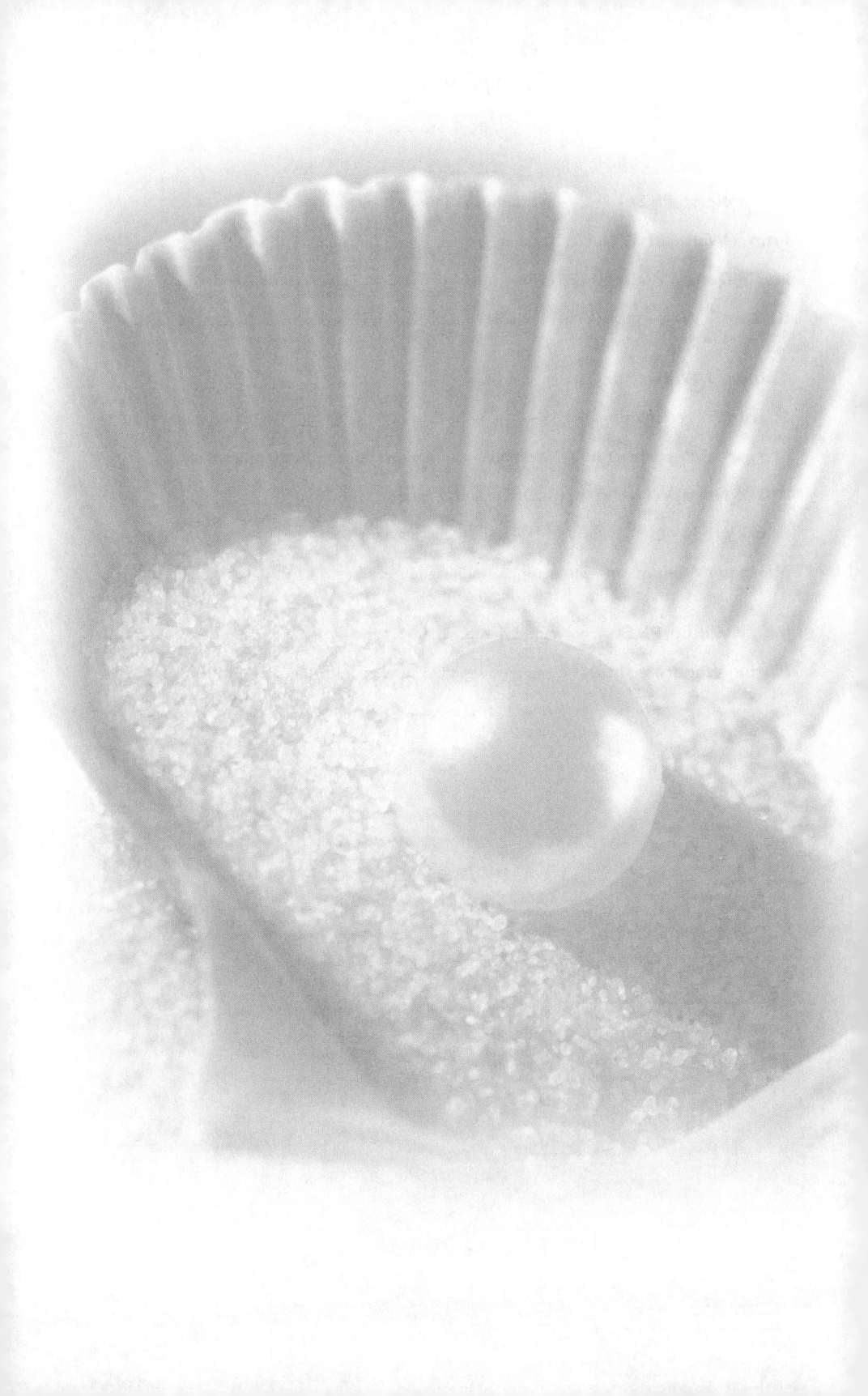

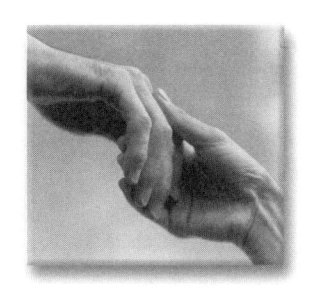

Contributor Index

A

Acts of the Apostles, 209
Adams, Henry, 219, 221
Aeschylus, 194
Al-Anon, 183
Alcoholics Anonymous, 163, 176, 190, 257
Alcott, Louisa May, 185
Alexander, Thea, 166
Ali, Muhammad, 257
Allen, Woody, 278
Alter, Robert and Jane, 26, 73
American Disabilities Act of 1990, 53
American Oxford Dictionary, 104
Amiel, Henri Frederic, 29, 131, 228
Analyze This, 179
Anamika, 249
Anderson, Carol, 51, 60
Andrim, Anna, 224
Angelou, Maya, 237, 248
Anthony, Susan B., 254
Apollinaire, Guillaume, 4
Aristotle, 180, 187, 207
Armstrong, Lance, 106, 107
Aronson, E., 58
As Good As It Gets, 250
Ash, Mary Kay, 177
Atwood, Margaret, 223
Augustine, Saint, 7, 104, 176, 280
Aurelius, Marcus, 35

B

Baba, Sai, 263
Bach, Marcus, 275
Bach, Richard, 9, 28, 281, 285
Bacon, Sir Francis, 107, 188
Balzac, Honoré de, 176
Barretta, Norma and Philip, 278, 279
Barrie, J. M., 189, 275
Barton, Bruce, 181
Bateson, Gregory, 30
Bateson, Mary Catherine, 122
Beasley, Joseph, 99
The Beatles, 272
Beckett, Samuel, 285
Beecher, Henry Ward, 165
Bell, Dr., 48
Ben-Gurion, David, 181
Bennett, E. A., 36
Bernard, Claude, 26
Berra, Yogi, 283
Bettelheim, Bruno, 201
Blake, William, 206
Blanton, Smiley, 180
Bolen, Jean Shinoda, 138
Bombeck, Erma, 46
Boone, Louis E., 198
Borge, Victor, 171
Borysenko, Joan, 37, 110, 128, 129, 263
Bourke-White, Margaret, 69
Bradbury, Ray, 169
Braden, Gregg, 269, 291, 293
Bradley, General Omar, 187
Bradshaw, John, 24
Branden, Nathaniel, 46
Bridges, Mondi, 8

Bridges, William, 4, 7, 125, 188, 226
Brilliant, Ashleigh, 132, 205
Brockovich, Erin, 83, 154, 167
Brontë, Charlotte, 229
Broude, Franklyn, 166
Brown, Rita Mae, 27
Browne, Sir Thomas, 259
Browning, Elizabeth Barrett, 251
Browning, Robert, 215
Buber, Martin, 214, 278
Buck, Pearl, 162, 223
Buddha, 112, 228, 229
Burgh, James, 116
Burns, George, 238
Butler, Samuel, 223
Byrd, Richard E., 121

C

Cabn, Edmond, 211
Campbell, Joseph, xvi, 35, 99, 124, 126, 133, 138, 139, 143, 155, 269, 273
Camus, Albert, 77, 225, 278
Canfield, Jack, 162
Capra, Fritjof, 20
Carlton, Richard, 112
Carlyle, Thomas, 145, 256
Carnegie, Dale, 170, 176
Carroll, Lewis, 262
Carter, Rosalynn, 17, 18, 22, 52, 87
Carter-Scott, Cherie, 156, 288
Casarjian, Robin, 237
Castaneda, Carlos, 157, 164, 199, 253
Cather, Willa, 237
Chaplin, Charlie, 124
Chávez, César, 274
Cher, 253
Chesterton, G. K., 6, 141, 145, 256
Chidvilasananda, Gurumayi, 260
Chou-Tun-I, 184
Christie, Agatha, 220, 249
Churchill, Winston, 107, 148, 150, 176, 188, 229
Cicero, xi
Cohen, Lilly, 57
Confucius, 38, 144
Consegrity Wellness Program, 4
Cooke, Alistair, 218

Corinthians, 239
Corr, Charles A., 88
Costin, Breck, 195, 260
Coty, Rene, 277
Coué, Emile, 262
A Course in Miracles, 194, 208
Cousins, Norman, 48, 60, 68, 181, 279
Croft, Roy, 239
Crosby, Greta W., 199
Crowley, Mary, 222
Cushing, Harvey, 171

D

Dalai Lama, 25, 107, 113, 151, 172, 206, 208, 217, 270, 287
Dannelley, Richard, 45
Dante Alighieri, 116, 289
Dass, Ram, 99, 119, 120, 127, 128, 234
Davies, Betty, 161
Davis, Elmer, 190
de Mille, Agnes, 227
Devlin, Bernadette, 190
Diagnostic and Statistical Manual of Mental Disorders (DSM-IV), xx, 44, 46, 49–50
Dickens, Rex, 109
Dickinson, Emily, 225
Dinesen, Isak, 161
Disraeli, Benjamin, 143, 223
Dix, Dorothea, 291, 293
Doka, Kenneth, 84
Donne, John, 275
Dossey, Larry, 110, 113, 261, 262, 271, 274, 275
Dostoevsky, Fyodor, 66
Drucker, Peter F., 204, 233
D'Souza, Alfred, 155, 271
DuBois, Charles, 187
Duff, Kat, 21, 66, 86, 91, 109, 119
Durkheim, Karlfried Graf, 145

E

Eccles, Sir John, 269
Eckhart, Meister, 129, 229
Edison, Thomas, 32, 149, 174
Einstein, Albert, 45, 77, 107, 153, 236, 248, 268
Eisenhower, Dwight David, 142, 147
Eldridge, Paul, 258

Eliade, Mircea, 105
Eliot, George, 232
Eliot, T. S., 5, 199, 236
Ellington, Duke, 31
Emerson, Ralph Waldo, 29, 32, 36, 60, 121, 148, 169, 190, 210, 216, 223, 229, 254, 268
Emmanuel, 186
Ephesians, 241
Epictetus, 114, 187, 250
Epicurus, 153
Eth, Spencer, 71
Euripedes, 184
Everett, William J., 66

F

Faraday, Michael, 273
Farrell, E., 48, 85
Federal Task Force on Homelessness and Mental Illness, 17
Fensterheim, Herbert, 142
Ferguson, Marilyn, 30, 125
Field, Johanna, 227
Figley, Charles R., 33, 52, 56, 57, 58, 59, 65, 67, 74, 83, 88, 94, 95, 191, 192, 234
Fisher, Roger, 232
Fitzgerald, F. Scott, 135
Flach, Frederic, 99, 197, 264
Fleming, Thomas, 165
Foch, Marshal Ferdinand, 26, 142
Ford, Henry, 66, 143, 222
Forrest Gump, 71, 248
Fortunato, John, 152
Fox, Matthew, 272
Francis of Assisi, Saint, 146, 291, 292
Frank, Anne, 215
Frank, Arthur, 56, 88, 162
Frankl, Viktor, 74, 122, 123, 129, 130, 160, 243, 255, 261, 269, 287
Franklin, Benjamin, 13, 175, 187, 210
French Foreign Legion, 281
Fromm, Erich, 124, 168, 180, 194
Frost, Robert, 140, 172, 176, 254
Fuller, Thomas, 170, 178

G

Galatians, 230
Galsworthy, John, 5

Gandhi, Mahatma, 110, 151, 166, 168, 231, 250, 252, 272
Gibb, Jack, 108
Gibbon, Edward, 142
Gibran, Kahlil, 115, 148, 269
Gide, André, 5, 7, 9, 123, 190, 280
Glascow, Arnold, 166
Goethe, Johann Wolfgang von, 26, 148, 163, 195, 199, 229, 257
Gold, Lois, 118, 121
Goldner, Diane, 272
Goldwyn, Sam, 37
Gottman, John, 235
Goulet, John, 284
Gracian, Baltasar, 224
Gravitz, Philip Benjamin, 90, 275
Gravitz, Sophie, 273, 283
Green, Hannah, 208
Greenberg, Rabbi Sidney, 167
Greiffe, Barrie Sanford, 207
Gretzky, Wayne, 166
Grissanti, Carl, 250
Grollman, Rabbi Earl A., 129, 149
Guest, Edgar A., 131
Gurudev (Yogi Amrit Desai), 22, 124

H

Halliday, Dr., 96
Hamlet, 51
Hansen, Mark Victor, 162
Harris, Bill, 155
Harris, Sydney, 247
Harvard Negotiation Project, 232–33
Hastings, James, 118
Hawking, Stephen, 188
Hei Hei, Rabbi Ben, 282
Hein, Piet, 276
Hellman, Lillian, 46
Hemingway, Ernest, 132
Hendrix, Harville, 35
Henry, Will, 189
Hepburn, Katherine, 185, 220
Herman, Judith, 67
Herron, Yolande D., 107
Heschel, Abraham, 15
Hesse, Herman, 117
Hill, Napoleon, 105, 211

Hillel, Rabbi, 192
Hippocrates, 60
Hoffer, Eric, 153
Hollen, John, 28
Holmes, Oliver Wendell, 165, 186, 275
Honda, Soichiro, 205
Hoover, Herbert, 186
Horace, 120, 256, 279
Horney, Karen, 238
Horowitz, Mardi Jon, 72
Houston, Jean, 99, 111, 112, 115, 116, 117, 118, 120, 241
Hubbard, Elbert, 212, 276
Hubbard, Ken, 286
Humphrey, Hubert H., 208
Hutchins, Robert M., 177
Huxley, Aldous, 108

I

Iacocca, Lee, 147
Ibn Gabirol, Shlomo, 212
I Ching, 152, 264
Illich, Ivan, 18, 219

J

Jackie Gleason Show, 152
James, William, 49, 54, 146, 169, 172, 206, 224
Jampolsky, Gerald, 186
Janoff-Bulman, Ronnie, 70
Jeans, Sir James, 182
Jefferson, Thomas, 25
Jesus, 162, 228, 234, 281
John, Book of, xi, 177
Johnson, Samuel, 31, 119, 203, 256
Johnson, Spencer, 269
Jordan, David Starr, 237, 257
Juan, Don, 108
Jung, Carl, 39, 99, 104, 122, 126, 133, 161, 196, 247, 253, 261, 281, 289

K

Kammann, Richard, 108
Kaplan, Rabbi Aryeh, 192
Karp, David A., 22, 23, 53, 75, 85, 87, 90, 94, 284
Kasl, Charlotte Davis, 34, 189
Kaslow, Florence, 25, 39

Kazantzakis, Nikos, 131
Keats, John, 111
Keller, Helen, 75, 115, 146, 167, 189, 226, 248
Kelly, James, 180
Kempton, Murray, 256
Kennedy, Joseph P., 176, 207
Kennedy, Robert, 204
Kerr, Jean, 276
Ketcham, Katherine, 19, 204, 216
Keyes, Ken, Jr., 119, 215
Kierkegaard, Soren, 25
King, Martin Luther, Jr., 30, 107, 164, 170, 172, 182, 209, 218, 231
Kipling, Rudyard, 180
Kissenger, Henry, 51
Kleinman, Arthur, 108
Koestler, Arthur, 168, 225
Kolk, Bessel A. van der, 69, 71, 72, 73
The Koran, 103, 114
Kreinheder, Albert, 109
Krugman, Steven, 73
Kübler-Ross, Elisabeth, 132, 238
Kurtz, Ernest, 204
Kushner, Rabbi Harold S., 37, 210, 211, 215, 263, 274, 286

L

Laing, R. D., 35
Lamers, William, Jr., 34
Lao Tzu, 137, 166, 191, 291, 292
Lauder, Estée, 149
Lawrence, D. H., 27
Le Guin, Ursula K., 222
Lerner, Max, 142
Lerner, Michael, 33
LeShan, Lawrence, 273
Levenson, Sam, 173
Levine, Michael, 31, 181
Levine, Stephen, 68, 218
Lewis, C. S., 23, 37, 140
Lincoln, Abraham, 67, 95, 167, 171, 210, 255
Lindbergh, Anne Morrow, 141, 165, 185
Lin Yutang, 184
London, Jack, 174
Longfellow, Henry Wadsworth, 6, 110
Lorde, André, 122
Love, Pat, 203

L

Lowell, James Russell, 216
Luke, Book of, 220
Luther, Martin, 106

M

Machado, Antonio, 120, 145
Machiavelli, Niccolò, 185
Maimonides, Moses, 178
Malachi, 116
Malloy, Merrit, 206
Mandela, Nelson, 155
Mansfield, Katherine, 197
Marsh, Diane, 17, 89
Marston, Ralph, 106
Maslow, Abraham, 38
Matthew, Book of, 162, 217
Maugham, W. Somerset, 179
Maurois, André, 214
May, Rollo, 126
McGrath, Mary Jo, 232
McKinnon, Dan, 179
McLaughlin, Mignon, 227
Mead, Margaret, 36
Meir, Golda, 178
Melville, Herman, 235
Mencken, H. L., 146
Mendelssohn, Moses, 215
Mental Health Policy Resource Center, 18
Merton, Thomas, 181, 240
Michelangelo, 115
Midrash Rabbah, 103
Milam, James, 19, 216
Miller, Arthur, 9, 193
Miller, Henry, 6, 113, 140
Milton, John, 171, 278
Mizner, Wilson, 8
Molière, Jean-Baptiste, 177
Montage, 69
Moore, Mary Tyler, 258
Moore, Thomas, 72
Moretta, Brenda, 57
Muller, Rev. Wayne, 23, 123, 217
Mumford, Ethel Watts, 253
Murphy, J., 48, 85
Myers, David G., 170, 206, 264, 284, 287

N

Napoleon, 138
National Association for Children of Alcoholics, 19
National Institute of Mental Health, 51
National Opinion Research Center, 214
Neimeyer, Robert A., 174
Nevelson, Louise, 128, 277
Newman, John Henry Cardinal, 9
Newton, John, 280
Niebuhr, Reinhold, 144
Nietzsche, Friedrich, 13, 72, 99, 114, 282
Nin, Anaïs, 26, 132, 141
Norwood, Sipreown, 260

O

Ogden, F., 114
Ordinary People, 72
Ornish, Dean, 210
Ortega y Gasset, José, 60

P

Parks, Rosa, 145
Pascal, Blaise, 145
Pasteur, Louis, 160
Patmore, Coventry, 193
Pavese, Cesare, 5
Peace Pilgrim, 175
Peale, Norman Vincent, 66, 146, 182
Pearsall, Paul, 34, 36, 76, 77, 265
Peck, M. Scott, 13, 36, 39, 99, 109, 154, 157, 163, 173, 192, 194, 216, 221, 235, 247, 250, 251, 255, 262, 279
Penn, William, 218
Peter, Lawrence J., 221, 255
Peters, Jon V., 204
Peters, Tom, 143
Phelps, Elizabeth Stuart, 277
Picasso, Pablo, 124, 150
Pierrakos, Eva, 117
Pines, A., 58
Pipher, Mary, 15, 22, 23, 35, 105, 167, 232, 247, 283, 286
Plato, 106, 251
Plautus, 173
Player, Gary, 148
Plutarch, 184

Pogo Possum, 37, 277
Pope, Alexander, 231
Post, Steve, 178
Primeau, Carol, 50
Procrustes, 26
Proust, Marcel, 119
Proverbs, Book of, xiii, 199
Psalms, 130, 197
Pynoos, Robert S., 71

R
Raines, Robert, 167
Rando, Therese A., 86
Redfield, James, 258, 261
Redstone, Sumner, 130
Reeve, Christopher, 143, 152
Register, Cheri, 21, 32
Rickenbacker, Eddie, 141
Ride, Sally, 142
Riemer, Rabbi Jack, 287
Riley, Pat, 154
Rilke, Rainer Maria, 137, 154, 287
Roberts, Bernadette, 127
Robertson, Frederick W., 117
Rockefeller, John D., Jr., 179
Rodgers, Pepper, 222
Rogers, Carl R., xx, 252
Rolland, John S., 47
Roosevelt, Eleanor, 172, 190, 224, 225
Roosevelt, Franklin D., 150, 151
Roosevelt, Theodore, 191
Rosenthal, A. M., 16
Roshi, Suzuki, 249
Rowell, Galen, 104
Rumi, Jalaluddin, 117, 139, 222
Runbeck, Margaret Lee, 140
Ruth, Babe, 177
Rutte, Martin, 209

S
Saadi, 173
Sacks, Oliver, 138
Sagan, Carl, 172, 286
Sa'ib of Tabriz, 29
Saint-Exupéry, Antoine de, 9, 146, 179, 211
St. James, Elaine, 16, 21, 171, 173
Sandberg, Carl, 259

Santayana, George, 228, 277
Saroyan, William, 240
Sarton, Mary, 205
Sartre, Jean-Paul, 161, 254
Satcher, David, 16
Satir, Virginia, 165, 227
Schaar, John, 291, 293
Schaefer, Eli J., 257
Schneerson, Rabbi Menachem, 213
Schuller, Robert H., 175, 182, 183
Schulstad, Mel, 20
Schwartz, Morrie, 21, 28, 76, 114, 171, 173, 195, 283
Schwartz, Tony, 157, 199
Schweitzer, Albert, 127, 170
Scott-Maxwell, Florida, 8, 125, 225
Secunda, Victoria, 18
Seligman, Martin, 89, 237
Seneca, 28, 113, 163, 259, 286
Senge, Peter, 205
Shakespeare, William, 45, 51, 76, 120, 212, 218
Shaw, Dr., 96
Shaw, George Bernard, 183, 205, 207, 217, 226, 227, 251
Sheehan, George, 278
Shin, Florence Scovel, 151
Siebert, Al, 103
Sills, Beverly, 147
Simmons, Annette, 160
Simonton, O. Carl, 68
Sittser, Gerald L., 74, 76, 98, 164
Skog, Susan, 16, 25
Small, Jacquelyn, 276
Smith, Huston, 263
Smith, Ron, 258
Solzhenitsyn, Alexander, 30, 224
Song of Solomon, 28
Sontag, Susan, 24, 53, 54
Sophocles, 169, 185, 219
Spock, Benjamin, 140
Star Wars, 189
Stevenson, Adlai E., 150
Stevenson, Robert Louis, 254, 260
Stone, Elizabeth, 222
Stone, W. Clement, 112
Stoppard, Tom, 5
Strong, Maggie, 83, 91, 93

Suzuki, Dr., 225
Swift, Jonathan, 53
Szent-Gyorgyi, Albert, 45

T

Tagore, Rabindranath, 6, 188
Talmud, 29, 121, 153, 212, 214, 288
Teilhard de Chardin, Pierre, 216
Telushkin, Rabbi Joseph, 204
Tennyson, Alfred Lord, 30, 104, 150
Teresa, Mother, 147, 151, 180, 209, 213, 215, 217, 264
Theresa of Lisieux, Saint, xiii
Thich Nhat Hanh, 261, 268, 271
Thomas à Kempis, 34, 164, 239
Thomsen, Robert, 129
Thoreau, Henry David, 220, 221, 223, 250, 278, 283
Thucydides, 208
Tillich, Paul, 212
Tolle, Eckhart, 270
Tolstoy, Leo, 168
Tomlin, Lily, 36
Topf, Linda Noble, 47, 139
Toynbee, Arnold J., 219
Truman, Harry, 219
Twain, Mark, 40, 145, 162, 187, 206, 230, 251

U

Underhill, Evelyn, 111
United Technologies Corporation, 285
Ury, William, 232

V

Valery, Paul, 6
Vasishtha, 118
The Vedas, 281
Vereen, Ben, 166
Viorst, Judith, 24, 27, 33, 270
Voltaire, 24, 68, 184
von Schiller, J. C. F., 168

W

Wagner, Richard, 259
Walker, Alice, 252
Walker, Harold, 183
Walsch, Neale Donald, 38, 239, 240, 291, 293
Walsh, Froma, 17, 20, 22, 34, 37, 51, 60, 96, 98, 191, 193, 194, 231
Walsh, Roger, 108
Washington, Booker T., 179, 186
Washington, Martha, 230
Watson, Dr., 48
Watson, Thomas J., Sr., 131
Webster's New Collegiate Dictionary, 65
Wegscheider, Sharon, 46, 47, 67, 249
Weil, Andrew, 130
Weller, Frances Ward, 221
Well Spouse Foundation, 86
Wheatley, Margaret, 259
White, T. H., 177
Whitehead, Alfred North, 253, 270
Wiesel, Elie, 161
Wilcox, Ella Wheeler, 208
Wilde, Oscar, 31, 116, 148, 154, 220
Williams, Carol, 57
Williamson, Marianne, 8, 27, 188, 271
Wilson, John P., 73
Wintle, Walter D., 280
Wittgenstein, Ludwig, 29
Wizard of Oz, 137
Woodman, Marion, 70
Woolis, Rebecca, 20, 84
Wordsworth, William, 213
Wright, Dr., 48
Wright, Steven, 230

Z

Zarienga, Peter, 169

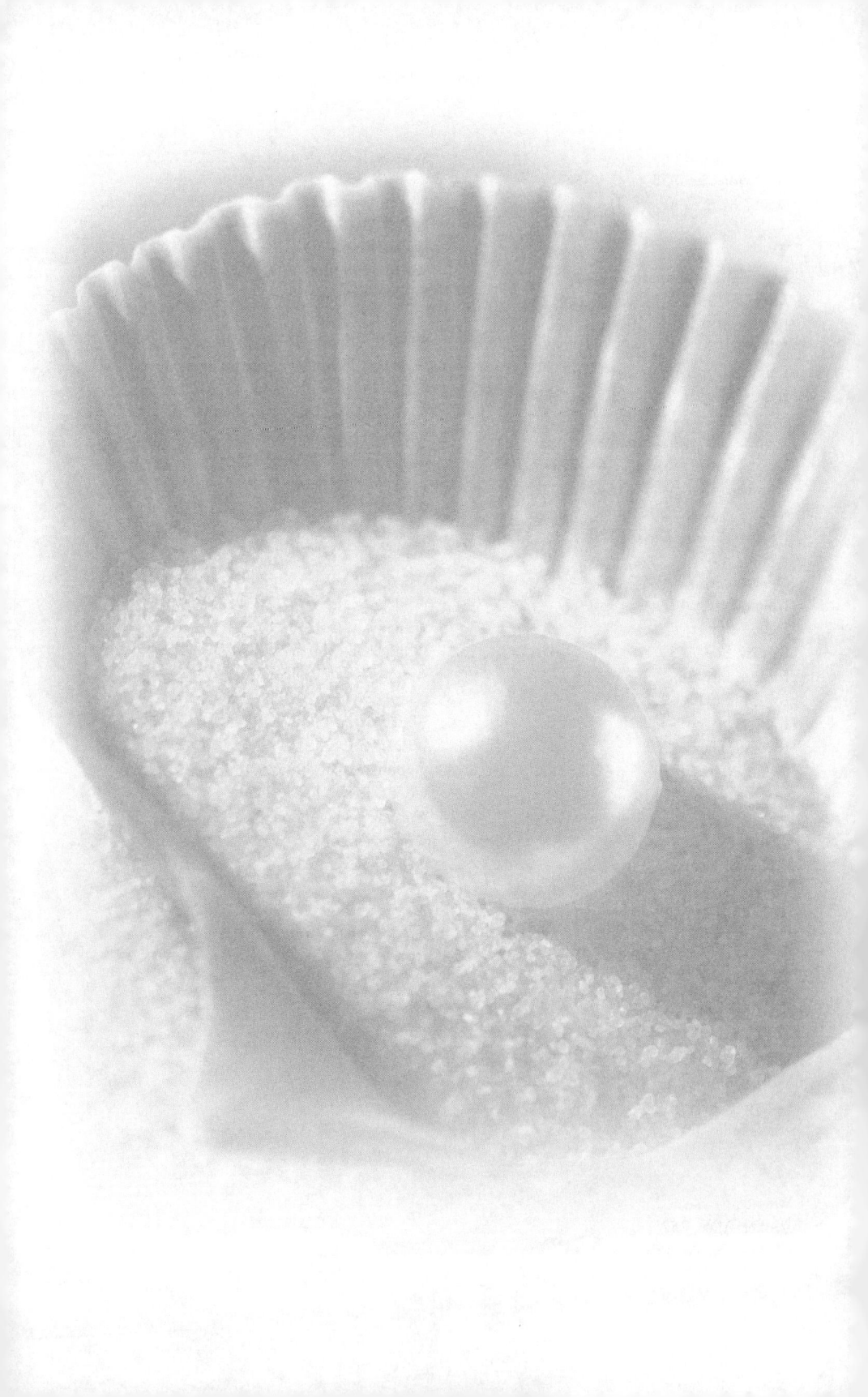

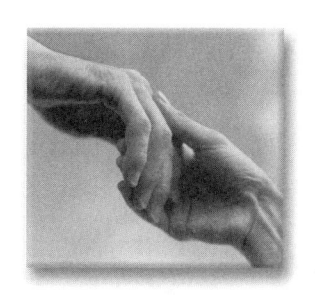

Subject Index

A

Abnormalities, 109
Abundance, 270
Abuse, 14, 68
Acceptance, 54, 172, 196–97, 250
Addiction. *See also* Alcoholism and alcohol abuse; Drug addiction
    effects of, 43, 47
    as a journey, 1–3, 10
    nature of, 34, 49
    occurring with illness and trauma, xii–xiii
    overcoming, 189
    prevalence of, 15
    types of, viii, 13–14
Adventures, 6, 142, 145
Adversity
    effects of, 103, 120
    increasing, vii
    kinds of, viii
    nature of, 112
    prevalence of, 21, 110
    as process, 1
    triumph and, viii, xiv, 132–33
Affection, 25, 179, 269
Age, 110, 228, 258
Alcoholism and alcohol abuse
    causes of, 20
    cost of, 16
    diagnosis of, 43
    effects of, 19, 20, 46, 69, 99
    families and, 67, 70, 78, 215, 216, 249
    prevalence of, 17, 19
    rehabilitation and, 165

ALS, 28, 114
Alzheimer's disease, 16, 57
Anger, 47, 164, 207, 239, 241
Anxiety, 165
Anxiety disorders, 51, 73
Arguments, 215, 216, 221
Assessment, 41, 42

B

Beauty, 32, 60, 132, 189, 282
Beginnings, 4–6, 8, 9, 291, 292
Beliefs, xii, 164, 262, 280
Betrayal, 118, 132–33
Bipolar disorder (manic depression), 18, 43, 49, 53
Blame, 28, 170, 193, 238, 251, 260
Brain disorders, 48
Bravery, 187, 190, 208, 227, 258. *See also* Courage
Burnout, 57, 58

C

Cancer, 8, 43, 48, 54, 69
Cardiovascular disease. *See* Heart disease
Caregiving, 55–60, 71, 72, 75, 86, 88, 96
Catastrophes, 65, 67
Change
    acceptance and, 196, 197
    fear of, 125
    freedom to, 269
    nature of, 8
    of oneself, 166, 195, 252, 257, 261, 288
    order and, 270

security and, 141
transition vs., 2, 7
Chaos, 2, 10, 42, 114
Charity, 178
Cheerfulness, 229–30
Children. *See also* Parenting
  abuse of, 14
  attitudes of, 95
  computers and, 16
  emotional health of, 97, 151
  fear of, 14
  hyperactive, 20
  losses and, 27
  reasons for having, 210, 222
  resilient, 191
Choices, 99, 125, 188
Commitment, 163, 175
Compassion, 179, 181, 199, 272
Compassion fatigue, 57
Compassion stress, 57, 59
Compulsions, 77
Conflict, 205
Confusion, 3, 6, 32, 42, 113
Conscious living, 293, 294
Contentment, 230, 257
Convenience, 225
Coping, 21, 70, 90, 159, 175, 183, 234
Courage. *See also* Bravery
  fear and, 141, 168, 187, 190, 251
  importance of, 173, 189, 193, 274
  love and, 191
  nature of, 39, 259
  need for, 165
  success and, 233
Creation, 9, 26, 139, 269
Creativity, 114, 173, 260
Crisis, 10, 96, 117, 135, 236
Cynicism, 232

D

Death, 27, 34, 68, 76, 250
Decisions, 55, 125, 160, 188, 212, 224, 233, 251
Denial, 32, 47, 69
Depression
  cure for, 232
  death and, 27
  definition of, 50
  disability and, 18
  nature of, 99
  prevalence of, 25
  stress and, 16
Diabetes, 21
Diagnosis
  advantages of, 41–43
  assessment vs., 41
  dual, 51
  family members and, 44, 47, 48, 55–60
  healing and, 61
  importance of, 40, 41, 44, 45–46, 53, 54–55, 61
  initial communication of, 47
  limitations of, 43
  replacement of person by, 51
Disability, 18, 22, 53, 57
Discipline, 163, 185, 195
Discovery, 40, 45, 160, 162, 190, 227
Dissipation, 259
Dissociation, 73
Distress, 17
Divorce, 27, 57
DNA, xiii
Doubt, 8, 182, 281
Dreams, 152, 175, 182
Drug addiction, 16, 17, 19, 20, 249. *See also* Substance abuse
Duty, 167, 223
Dysthymic disorder, 50, 73

E

Embarrassment, 32
Emergencies, viii
Emotions
  importance of, 126, 189
  negative, 60
Encouragement, 168
Endings, 5–6, 9, 291
Enlightenment, 112, 247
Entropy, 77
Excellence, 143
Expectations, 91, 188, 238, 287
Experience, 108, 258

F

Facts, 160
Failure
  fear of, 177, 198
  inevitability of, 284
  nature of, 152
  power and, 188
  success and, 130, 175, 196, 205
  wisdom and, 240
Faith
  absence of, 183
  doubt vs., 8
  importance of, 167, 168, 263
  nature of, 7, 182, 183, 280
  power of, 167, 183
  tests of, 128
  understanding and, 176
Families. *See also* Refamilying
  alcoholism and, 67, 70, 78, 215, 216, 249
  crisis and, 96
  diagnosis and, 44, 47, 48, 55–60
  happy, 200, 203, 238, 242, 283
  importance of, 203, 205–6, 207, 235
  mental illness and, 51, 85, 87, 89
  neglect of, 20, 22, 34, 36, 267, 284
  problems and, 201–2
  strong, 200
  in today's world, 39
  training vs. blaming, 37, 82, 193, 209
  traumatized, 33, 58, 74, 88, 89
  wounds and, 78, 81–83
Fear
  absence of, 24, 26, 142
  of change, 125
  courage and, 141, 168, 187, 190, 251
  of failure, 177, 198
  freedom and, 30
  nature of, 28, 68, 110, 142, 186
  of new experiences, 27
  origins of, 36
  overcoming, 150, 164, 169, 170, 194
  of potential, 38
  source of, 249
  of suffering, 69
  of trying, 175
Forgiveness, 169, 170, 194, 231, 234, 237
Fortitude, 188

Fragmentation, 65
Freedom, 25, 30, 122, 190, 195, 199, 218, 254, 255
Friends, 153, 177, 210, 218, 220–22, 252–55
Future, the, 154, 225, 226, 282, 293

G

Genius, 166, 224
Giving, 178, 179, 180, 209, 211, 213, 220
Giving up, 32, 33, 89, 208, 229
God
  actions of, 151, 153, 161, 164, 168, 186
  belief in, 37, 184
  communication with, 36
  existence of, 23, 229
  justice and, 106
  nature of, 276
  praying to, 150
  worship of, 253
Gossip, 26
Grace, 127, 128, 280
Gratitude, 173
Greatness, 109, 171, 181, 204, 227
Grief
  American approach to, 34
  effects of, 117, 144, 149
  nature of, 84, 129, 174
  perspective and, 262
  shared, 238
Grudges, 234
Guilt, 64, 76, 98

H

Habits, 164, 177
Hallucinations, 50
Happiness
  at home, 203
  nature of, 108, 115, 140, 170, 180, 187, 225, 230, 238, 260, 277
  source of, 127, 141, 226, 264, 269, 284, 286
  truth and, 242
Hatred, 164, 208
Healing
  choices and, 99
  diagnosis and, 61
  primary determinants of, 78–79

refamilying and, 202–3, 240–43
Health, 261, 274, 275, 284
Health care, 21, 40
Heart disease, 21, 25, 174
Heaven, 118, 126, 169, 278
Hell, 26, 66, 126, 278, 289
Heroes, xvii, 124, 135–36, 143–44, 154–55, 158, 190, 278
Home, 136–37, 158, 202–4, 211
Homelessness, 17
Honesty, 199
Hope, 22, 30–31, 181, 182, 193, 194, 276, 279
Hospice, 34
Hugs, 165, 209
Hyperactivity, 20
Hypertension, 20

I

Ideals, 215
Ignorance, 36
Illness. *See also individual illnesses*
  early stages of, 32
  effects of, 43, 86, 108
  health and, 261
  as a journey, 1–3, 10, 139
  occurring with addiction and trauma, xii–xiii
  prevalence of, 15, 21, 24, 66
  social context of, 39–40
  stigmatization and, 63, 76, 77, 119
  types of, viii, 13
  value of, 68, 86
Imagination, 9
Impossibility, 138, 145, 262
Inconvenience, 6
Information explosion, 14
Initiation, 136
Insanity, 27
Inspiration, 174
Interdependence, 181, 217, 235, 275
Isolation, 23

J

Journeys, 1–3, 10, 135–39, 145, 152, 157–58, 200, 289
Joy, 221, 226, 229, 238, 259
Justice, 106, 145

K

Kindness, 151, 180, 214, 282
Knowledge, 268

L

Laughter, 171
Leadership, 219
Learning, 26, 212, 213, 245–46, 272, 285
Learning disabilities, 20
Learning strategies, 159
Lessons, 107, 110, 156, 245–46
Life
  growth opportunities in, xvii, 40
  meaning and, 76, 78, 103, 122, 129, 151, 157, 160, 161, 195, 284
  nature of, 8, 9, 22, 24, 29, 36, 40, 78, 108, 112, 123, 124, 125, 130, 138, 148, 151, 155, 199, 226, 229, 254, 260, 263, 268, 271, 275, 282
  pain and, 13
  trauma and, 74
Limitations, 28, 106
Listening, 212
Love
  giving and, 213
  hatred and, 208
  importance of, 30, 66, 211, 232, 272
  nature of, 173, 177, 180, 188, 206, 213, 215, 220, 222, 223, 239, 251
  pain and, 69
  power of, 164, 167, 186, 191, 210, 213, 216, 218, 219, 237, 271, 272
  truth and, 228
  work and, 148
Lupus, 21, 54

M

Manic depression. *See* Bipolar disorder
Marriage, 91, 96, 214, 235
Maturity, 253
Mental growth, 36, 39, 247
Mental illness. *See also individual illnesses*
  American Disabilities Act and, 53
  brain disorders and, 48
  caregivers and, 69, 75
  cost of, 16
  effects of, 22

families and, 51, 85, 87, 89
medications for, 52
with other problems, 20
prevalence of, 16, 17, 18
stigma of, 20, 53
types of, 44
Mentoring, 231
Miracles, 7, 149, 181, 186, 237
Moderation, 184
Mourning, 75, 76
Multiple sclerosis, 21
Music, 173
Mystics, 35, 49, 113
Mythology, 139

N
Narcissism, 232
Nature, 73
Negotiation, 232–33
Neurosis, 116, 281
9/11 attacks, 14

O
Obedience, 256
Obsessive-compulsive disorder (OCD), 18, 24, 43, 49
Obstacles, 66, 107, 155, 157, 185
Odysseus, 126, 137, 202
Openness, 194
Opportunity, 10, 31, 107, 114, 149, 176, 272, 277
Optimism, 31, 144, 176

P
Pain
  beauty and, 132
  causes of, 35, 38
  feeling, 72
  importance of, 32, 106, 113, 154, 167
  love and, 69
  nature of, 18, 114, 115
  prevalence of, 13, 15, 23, 104, 262
Paradox, 3
Parenting, 35, 221
Parkinson's disease, 43
Patience, 151, 173
Peace
  inner, 175, 288
  nature of, 217, 261
Perseverance, 104, 119, 147, 149, 152, 163
Personality disorder, 50
Pessimism, 31, 144, 176, 279
Pity, 111
Post-traumatic stress disorder (PTSD), 46, 52, 58, 70, 71, 192
Poverty, 286
Power, 188, 219, 268
Powerlessness, 33
Prayer, 7, 36, 150, 176, 198, 199
Prejudice, 24, 40, 250
Primary sufferers
  impact on, 43, 81
  secondary vs., xvii–xviii
  stigmatization of, 81
Problems
  in bunches, xii–xiii, 10–11
  causes of, 38
  diagnosis of, 40, 41–44
  families and, 201–2
  growth and, 36, 39
  nature of, 29, 45, 192, 236, 275, 289
  prevalence of, 15
  side effects of, 43
  types of, 14–15, 39
Psychology, sacred, 111, 120
Psychosis, 43, 50, 51

Q
Quantum science, 293

R
Reality, 78, 131, 140, 270
Recovery, 46, 84
Recrimination, 60
Refamilying, 202–3, 238, 240–43
Relationships, 38, 204, 206, 207
Remorse, 60
Renewal, 4, 103
Resentment, 60
Resilience, 96, 191, 197, 264, 267, 286
Responsibility, 37, 186, 273
Returning, 136–37, 158, 202

S

Schizophrenia, 18, 20, 35, 36, 49, 50, 51
Secondary sufferers
   impact on, 43, 55, 82, 83–98
   neglect of, 43, 56, 81–82
   number of, 81
   primary vs., xvii–xviii
   stigmatization of, 82
Secondary traumatic stress (STS), 58, 71
Security, 25, 141, 248
Self-confidence, 108
Self-esteem, 252
Separation, 136
Serenity, 280, 287
Sex, 90, 214, 278
   Shame
   illness and, 61, 64, 76, 77
   nature of, 24
   victims and, 67
Skepticism, 183
Smiling, 171, 209
Sorrow, 129, 161, 221, 229, 249
Soulmaking, 111, 116, 120, 241
Spirit, 228, 274
Spiritual growth, 36, 39, 173, 247
Strength, 255
Stress, 16, 71, 72, 109, 192, 193, 234. See also Compassion stress; Post-traumatic stress disorder; Secondary traumatic stress
Substance abuse, 51, 73. See also Addiction; Drug addiction
Success
   courage and, 233
   definition of, 265
   failure and, 130, 175, 196, 205
   measuring, 207, 208
   nature of, 166, 171, 178, 195, 205, 280
   work and, 162
Suffering
   causes of, 25, 37, 38, 155
   effects of, 105, 113, 116, 117, 154, 185, 278
   ending, 162
   enlightenment and, 112
   fear of, 69
   inauthentic, 133
   intolerance for, 22
   meaning and, 122, 123, 129, 130
   nature of, 77, 119
   prevalence of, 15, 23, 75, 113, 262
Suicide, 16, 19, 74, 95
Support groups, 196
Surprise, 60
Survivors
   guilt of, 98
   victims vs., 67
Sympathy, 25

T

Teaching, 119, 219, 285
Temptation, 211
Terrorism, 14
Thought, 265, 294
Thresholds, 10
Time, 105
Tolerance, 172, 255
Tragedy, 65, 110, 121, 129, 246, 260, 274
Transitions, 2, 3, 7
Trauma
   causes of, 69, 71
   consistency of, 72
   effects of, 73, 74
   encoding of, 95
   as a journey, 1–3, 10
   long-term adjustment to, 73
   occurring with addiction and illness, xii–xiii
   pathology and, 70
   prevalence of, 15
   side effects of, 43
   social support and, 71
   types of, viii
Triumph, viii, xiv, 132–33, 240
Trust, 186
Truth(s)
   denial and, 69
   eternal, xii–xiii, xiv
   happiness and, 242
   love and, 228
   nature of, 30, 46, 59, 105, 175, 177, 269, 280, 281
Twelve-step programs, 163

U

Understanding, 60, 131, 146, 172, 176, 228, 277

V

Vacations, 174
Valor, 259
Values, 20, 22, 34
Victims, 67, 70, 74, 260, 284
Violence, 14, 35
Virtue, 237, 257

W

Wealth, 284, 286
Wisdom
   age and, 258
   nature of, 153, 184, 185, 186, 206, 212, 214, 224, 225, 237, 257
   source of, 39, 130, 157, 240, 276
Wonder, 60, 160
Words, power of, ix, xi–xii
Work, 148, 149, 162, 231, 247
World Trade Center, 14
Wounds
   acceptability of, 63
   deep, 64–65, 79
   effects of, 78, 81–83, 101–3, 121
   as journeys, 135–37
   multiple, 61, 64
   profane, 101–2, 103, 125
   sacred, 102–3, 117, 118, 121
   types of, 63–64, 101–3
   unavoidable, 99

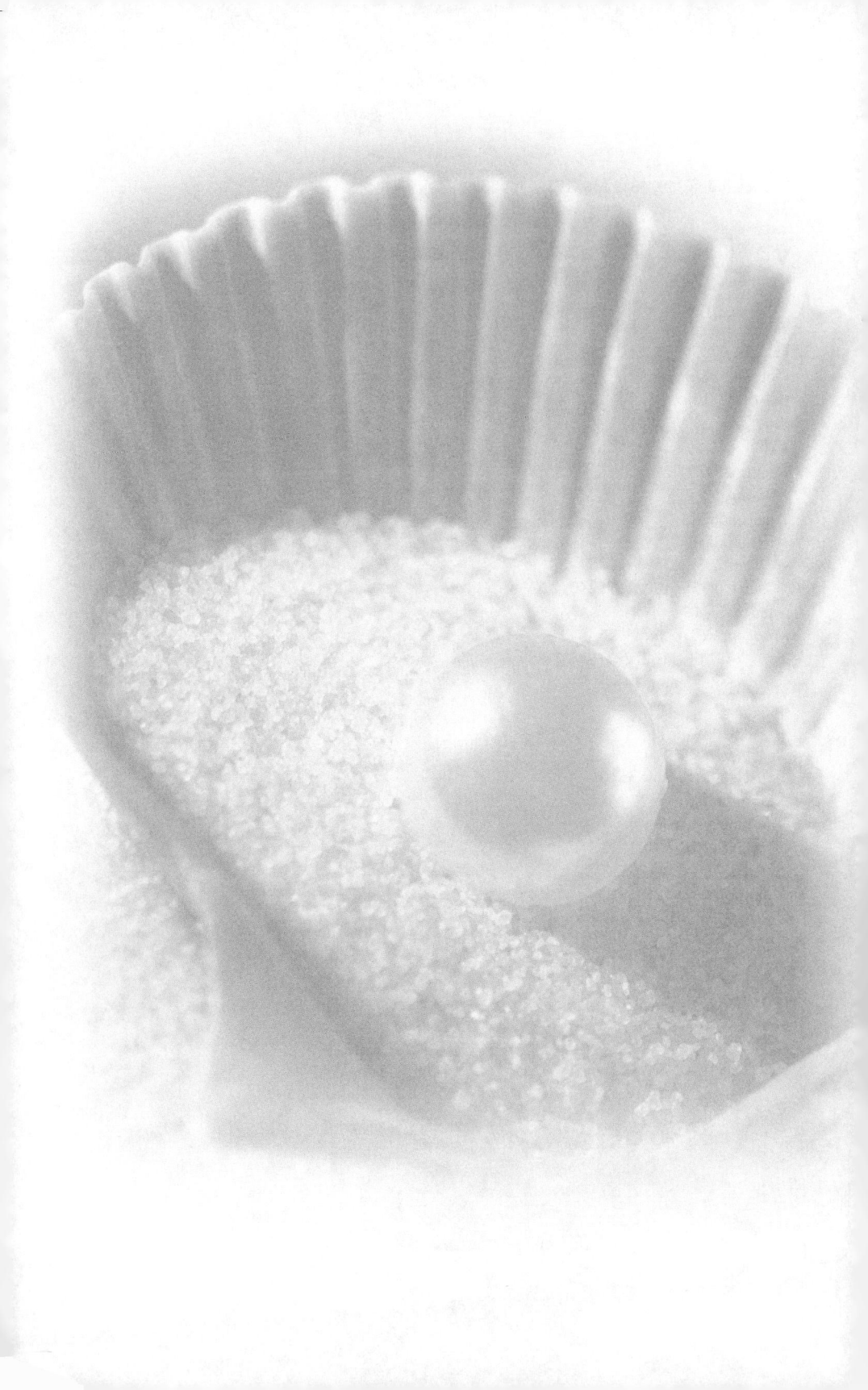

Quick Order Form

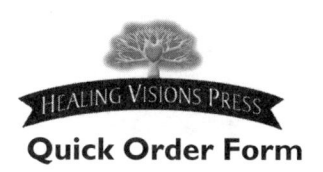

Online orders   www.HealTheFamily.com
Fax orders   805-543-5160
Telephone orders   800-718-7080 or 805-545-8398
E-mail orders   orders@HealTheFamily.com
Postal orders   Healing Visions Press
         P.O. Box 4035
         San Luis Obispo, CA 93403

I would like to order additional copies of *Facing Adversity: Words That Heal* at $24.95 each (see below).

For quantity discounts and special sales, please go to orders@HealTheFamily.com or call 800-718-7080.

If you found this book helpful, you might be interested in the following from Healing Visions Press:

Quantity	Item	Total Price
_____	*Facing Adversity: Words That Heal* @$24.95	_____
_____	*Mental Illness and the Family: Unlocking the Doors to Triumph* @$24.95	_____
_____	*Obsessive Compulsive Disorder: New Help for the Family* @$21.95	_____
	Sales tax	_____
	(Please add 7.75% for books shipped to CA addresses)	
	Shipping & handling	_____
	($5 for the first book and $3 for each additional book)	
	Total Due	_____

Name _____

Address _____

City _____

State _____ Zip _____

Telephone _____ E-Mail address _____

Payment ____Check *(Make checks payable to Healing Visions Press)*
             ____Visa ____MasterCard

Card number _____

Name on card _____ Exp. Date _____

Thank you for your order!
Please visit our website at www.HealTheFamily.com

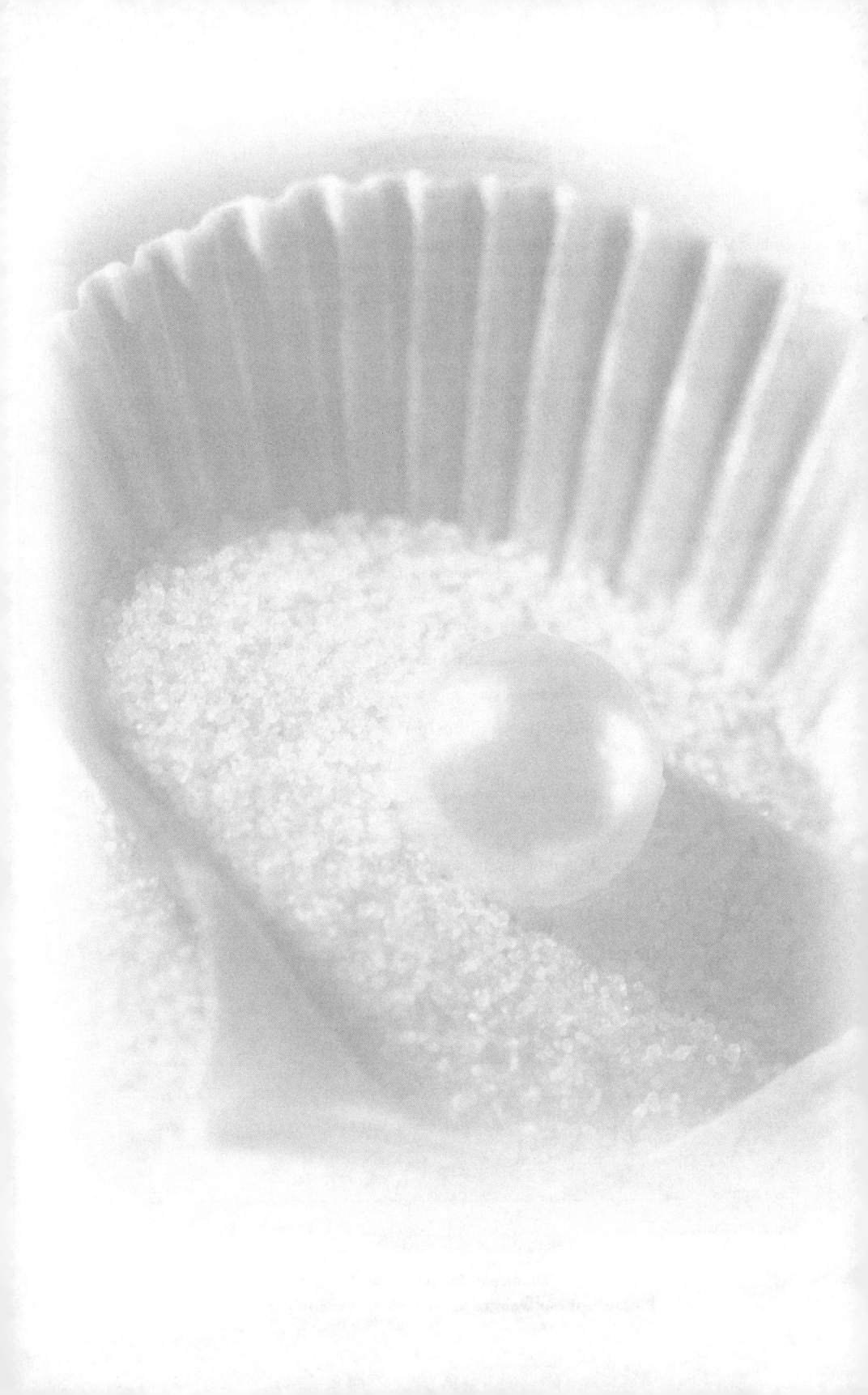

HEALING VISIONS PRESS

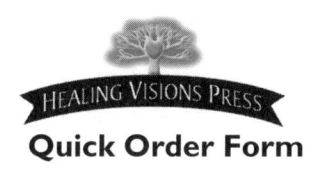

Quick Order Form

Online orders	www.HealTheFamily.com
Fax orders	805-543-5160
Telephone orders	800-718-7080 or 805-545-8398
E-mail orders	orders@HealTheFamily.com
Postal orders	Healing Visions Press
	P.O. Box 4035
	San Luis Obispo, CA 93403

I would like to order additional copies of *Facing Adversity: Words That Heal* at $24.95 each (see below).

For quantity discounts and special sales, please go to orders@HealTheFamily.com or call 800-718-7080.

If you found this book helpful, you might be interested in the following from Healing Visions Press:

Quantity	Item	Total Price
_____	*Facing Adversity: Words That Heal* @$24.95	_____
_____	*Mental Illness and the Family: Unlocking the Doors to Triumph* @$24.95	_____
_____	*Obsessive Compulsive Disorder: New Help for the Family* @$21.95	_____
	Sales tax	_____
	(Please add 7.75% for books shipped to CA addresses)	
	Shipping & handling	_____
	($5 for the first book and $3 for each additional book)	
	Total Due	_____

Name _____

Address _____

City _____

State _____ Zip _____

Telephone _____ E-Mail address _____

Payment ____Check *(Make checks payable to Healing Visions Press)*

____Visa ____MasterCard

Card number _____

Name on card _____ Exp. Date _____

Thank you for your order!
Please visit our website at www.HealTheFamily.com

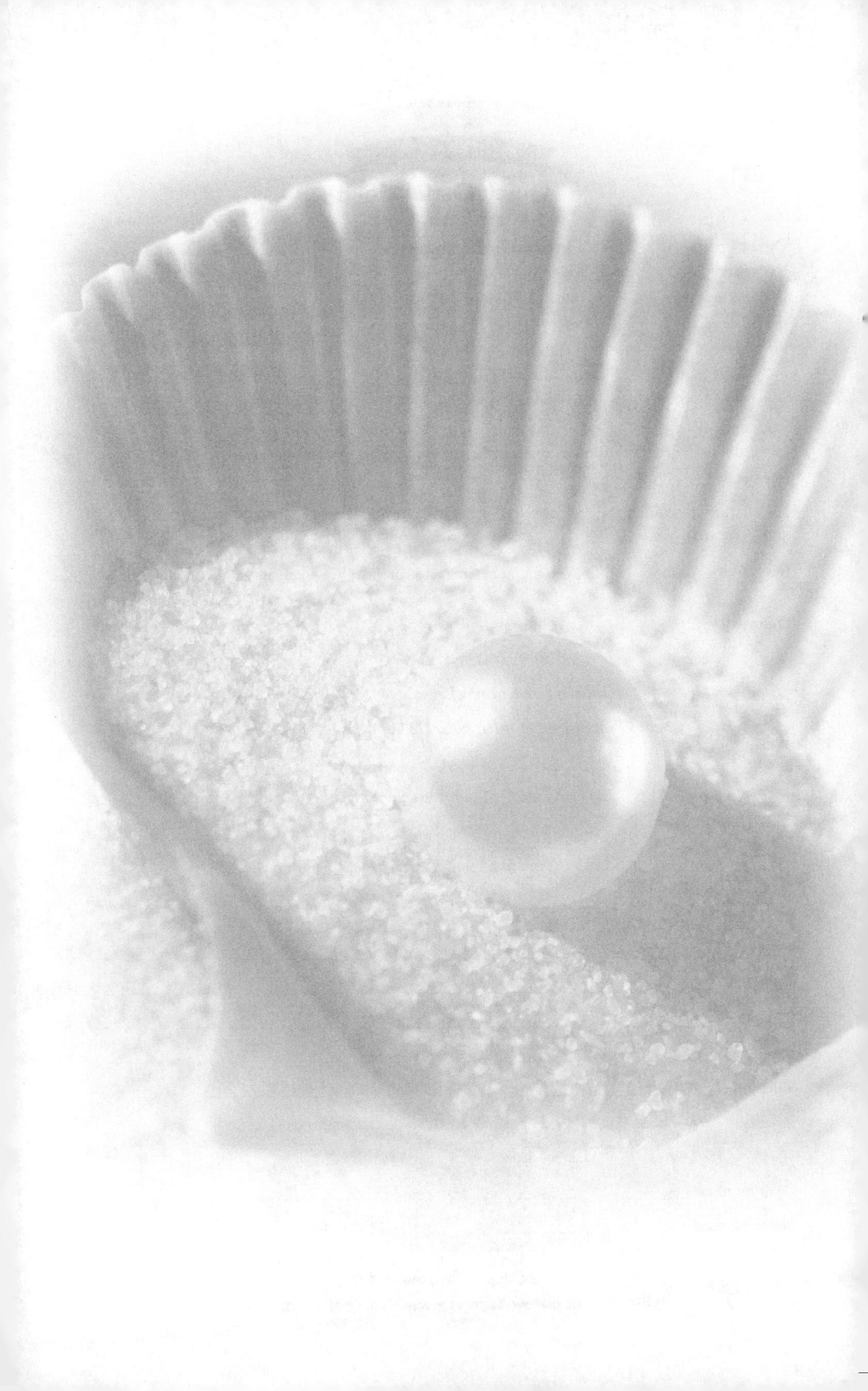

Quick Order Form

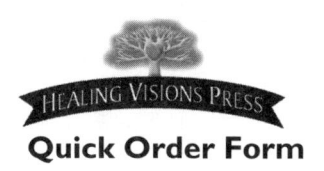

Online orders   www.HealTheFamily.com
Fax orders   805-543-5160
Telephone orders   800-718-7080 or 805-545-8398
E-mail orders   orders@HealTheFamily.com
Postal orders   Healing Visions Press
                     P.O. Box 4035
                     San Luis Obispo, CA 93403

I would like to order additional copies of *Facing Adversity: Words That Heal* at $24.95 each (see below).

For quantity discounts and special sales, please go to orders@HealTheFamily.com or call 800-718-7080.

If you found this book helpful, you might be interested in the following from Healing Visions Press:

Quantity	Item	Total Price
_____	*Facing Adversity: Words That Heal* @$24.95	_____
_____	*Mental Illness and the Family: Unlocking the Doors to Triumph* @$24.95	_____
_____	*Obsessive Compulsive Disorder: New Help for the Family* @$21.95	_____
	Sales tax	_____
	(Please add 7.75% for books shipped to CA addresses)	
	Shipping & handling	_____
	($5 for the first book and $3 for each additional book)	
	Total Due	_____

Name _____

Address _____

City _____

State _____   Zip _____

Telephone _____   E-Mail address _____

Payment ____Check *(Make checks payable to Healing Visions Press)*
              ____Visa   ____MasterCard

Card number _____

Name on card _____   Exp. Date _____

Thank you for your order!
Please visit our website at www.HealTheFamily.com

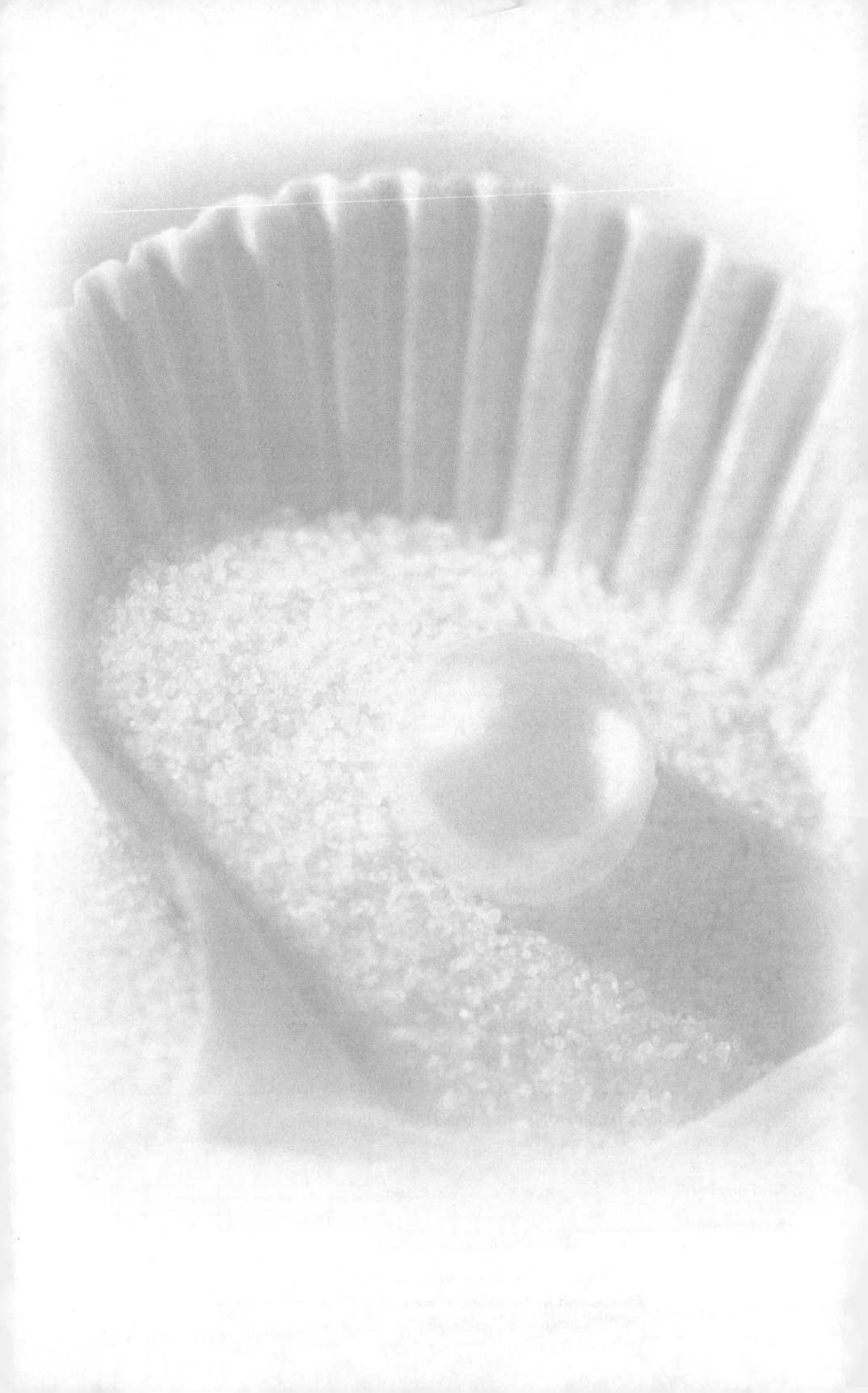